Lara Moore

Intermittent Fasting for Women 101

The Only Step-by-Step Guide for Weight Loss, Even If You Are Over 50, with the Keto Diet and Self-Cleansing Through the Metabolic Process of Autophagy.

Table of Contents

Introduction

Welcome to the valuable reading journey found in *Intermittent Fasting for Women 101*, Thank you for your purchase.

Intermittent fasting is a method of eating that any woman can use to lose weight and achieve a healthier body. Unlike with traditional fasting, intermittent fasting allows you to cycle between periods of eating and not eating and does not restrict you to a strict process. Doing so, it activates a biological process called autophagy. This process cleans out the toxins from your cells. When triggered by intermittent fasting, as well as other methods such as the keto diet and exercise, autophagy slowly gets you habituated into healthier lifestyle habits like eating nutritious foods and exercising.

This book doesn't skip a beat in telling you how to make intermittent fasting a seamless part of your life. The book even covers topics like how pregnant women and women over 50 can successfully start intermittent fasting. Read on to change how you look and feel for the better.

Most people get interested in intermittent fasting and autophagy because of what these processes can do for their weight through natural detox. While these benefits are something you don't want to miss out on, the astounding thing is that intermittent fasting can do even more for you. When we talk about the many positive effects intermittent fasting has on your body, we can split them into two categories: effects that you see fairly soon and long-term effects that mean permanent positive changes in the grand scheme of things.

The effects that you see early on include younger-looking skin with a glow, and an increase in the energy for higher productivity every day. These alone usually convince people that they should do intermittent fasting to trigger autophagy, but there is even more it can do for them. This advanced process causes all the operations in your body to run much more smoothly. This leads to positive effects like less inflammation, lower cholesterol, lowered risk of developing cancer, lowered risk of developing heart disease, and a massive reduction in the knots and tangles in the brain linked to neurodegenerative diseases like Alzheimer's disease and Parkinson's disease.

It would be hard to decide which effects to your health you care about most, but fortunately, there is no need for you to choose. If you follow the effective routine of intermittent fasting, you will gain all of these benefits and more. Luckily, this book has everything you need to know about how to get started intermittent fasting painlessly and without a misstep.

Again, I say thank you for choosing to read this book! Every effort was made to ensure it is full of as much useful information as possible. Turn the page and let's get started nourishing your mind for the benefit of your body!

Chapter 1 - The Modern Woman and Weight Loss

"The philosophy of fasting calls upon us to know ourselves, to master ourselves, and to discipline ourselves, the better to free ourselves. To fast is to identify our dependencies and free ourselves from them."
- Tariq Ramadan

The desire to lose weight is very common among American women. However, weight loss typically goes hand in hand with other changes that they desire for their bodies. Luckily, intermittent fasting has been proven by scientific research to spur weight loss in women of all ages that were studied. Its health benefits were also shown to extend far beyond weight loss. If you want to feel more energetic, lower your risk of developing heart disease, and reduce inflammation, intermittent fasting is the one sure lifestyle change that will accomplish all these feats and more.

In the four years between 2013 and 2016, half of American citizens said that they wanted to lose weight. You are not alone. Many people want to shed unwanted pounds. Studies show that more women than men want to implement lifestyle choices that will allow them to lose weight.

While approximately 60% of women said they had put effort into losing weight, only about 40% of men said the same thing. Moreover, age factors into the equation too. Approximately 43% of adults over 60 want to lose weight. The percentage is different in other age groups. About 50% of adults between the ages of 20 years and 39 years want to lose weight. The biggest percentage falls into the 40 to 59 year age group with more than 52%.

These results ranged across other demographic criteria such as race, income, education, and more. It was also found that the more results a person gains with weight loss, the more likely that this person is to continue with their weight loss journey.

People who want to lose weight employ all sorts of techniques to achieve this purpose. The most commonly used techniques are dieting and exercise. These techniques are so common because of their effectiveness and their necessity for maintaining good health of mind and body. At no point will you see advice against the use of diet and exercise. Rather, it will be stressed how important it is for you to maintain a good diet and exercise routine in conjunction with intermittent fasting.

There is a mountain of evidence to suggest that, to compound the weight loss effects of diet and exercise, practicing intermittent fasting is your best bet. This is because intermittent fasting triggers autophagy. Luckily, you do not have to take my word for this. I will continue to cite scientific research to back up the material written in this book so you can rest assured. You can also browse the appendix of studies included at the back of the book.

The best part is that intermittent fasting requires little change to your day-to-day life when compared to other techniques. Women all of the globe have a lot on their plates in their daily lives. Therefore, using a weight loss technique that adds as little to their to-do list is essential and practical.

The practicality of intermittent fasting also makes it more likely that the faster will follow through with the process, instead of quitting shortly after starting the way that many women do with rigid weight loss practices. Many other methods demand that the practitioner implement drastic new measures to already hectic routines. These demands make it highly likely that most people will not stick to the new routine.

Make it easy for you to lose those unwanted pounds without ridiculous changed to your full life. Intermittent fasting is that easy choice that keeps life simple while still allowing you to lose weight.

Remember that intermittent fasting without the implementation of a proper diet and exercise routine will not gain you the results that you want. In fact, it can cause negative consequences, one of which can be weight gain. Both proper diet and exercise are necessary for achieving an advanced stage of autophagy.

The coming chapters will expand on the definition of intermittent fasting, the benefits you can expect to get from practicing it, the different methods of intermittent fasting and how to choose the right method of intermittent fasting for you and your lifestyle. Let's get you started with a basic idea of intermittent fasting works first.

Intermittent fasting is the practice of alternating between periods eating ("feasting") and not eating ("fasting"). There are a lot of ways this can be done, but a simple way is to choose a fixed period of time that you will fast every day. Beginners typically start with a minimum fasting period of 5 hours then build on the number of hours of fasting as they grow more comfortable with the process.

Women who start intermittent fasting with this simple method normally commit to not eating between the hours of 1 p.m. and 6 p.m. every day. The normal progression of this is to add more fasting hours after about one month. Therefore, she will have a 7-hour fast and start fasting earlier in the day or end the fast period later in the day. She will progressively build on her fast hours with the reasonable goal of reaching a 12-hour fast period.

This routine does not change her lifestyle much apart from small changes to her eating schedule. Despite this small amount of change, she will notice huge changes in the health of her body and mind. With almost no effort and a powerful strategy, she will lose weight and unlock numerous other positive effects on her body.

That woman can be you.

A Broad Look at the Weight Loss Challenges Faced by Modern Women

So far, we have explained the reason why intermittent fasting (often shortened to IF) is the perfect solution for you if you want to make your body look and feel healthier with minimal changes to your lifestyle.

Women tend to have more difficulty losing weight compared to their male counterparts. This is why I *just* had to make this information on intermittent fasting available to women no matter their race, age or any other demographic information. Intermittent fasting is the strategy that can level the weight loss playing field with men for women.

As exciting as the prospect of effective weight loss is for women everywhere, intermittent fasting should be approached in the right manner for the results to be worthy of the strategy. Intermittent should *always* be supported with an equally effective diet and exercise routine. I will continue to stress this fact time and time again throughout this book because it is such an important fact that you must drill into your head and implement in reality. Intermittent fasting should not be practiced in singularity.

In keeping with an effective diet and exercise routine, there are a few rules that women must abide by to ensure they get the best weight loss results from intermittent fasting. First, a woman trying to slim down needs to take in fewer calories than she is consuming. This is simple math. You cannot afford to gorge yourself on calories, especially by consuming lots of sugary and fatty foods, and expect that your waistline will get smaller just because you limit that consumption to a specific window in the day. This practice just will not add up.

Secondly, intermittent fasting needs to be supported by eating the right foods. Even if you eat fewer calories, if you getting them from the wrong sources like refined sugars and carbs, and saturated fats, intermittent fasting is still unlikely to help you shed the unwanted pounds. Instead, you need to source calories from foods that have good nutritional value like vitamins and minerals, and not just empty. These are foods like fatty fish, whole grains low in carbs, nuts, non-starchy vegetables, some fruit, leafy greens, and more.

Many people, even men, encounter difficulty when trying to eat healthier. But being more mindful of how the food that you eat affects your body goes a long way in helping you make better eating choices. Besides, with the right seasoning and preparation, you can make almost any food pleasing to your palette. You just need to be creative.

The third rule you need to follow to get the most benefit from intermittent fasting is to practice physical activity daily and to have a weekly exercise routine. Common physical activities that are great to practice in daily life include walking instead of driving or taking the elevator when you can and doing chores like sweeping.

It is recommended that adults should get at least 150 minutes of moderate or 75 minutes of vigorous aerobic activity very week. Aerobic exercises help get your heart pumping and help you lose weight in addition to gaining you several other health benefits like decreased risk of developing cardiovascular diseases. Luckily, you do not need to get a gym membership to incorporate aerobic exercise into your weekly routine. Examples of simple moderate aerobic exercises that you can do at home or on your own include walking, jogging and swimming. Even mowing the lawn and gardening can get you a good moderate aerobic exercise session. Running is an example of vigorous aerobic exercise.

Weekly aerobic exercise sessions need to be coupled with strength training to build and keep muscle strength. For the best results, an adult needs to get at least 2 weekly session of this type of exercise of 12 to 15 repetitions in each session. The use of weight machines and resistance tubes can be used in strength training. But you do not have to get fancy. The use of your own body weight is great for strength training. That is why pushups are such a popular exercise.

Other rules that you should follow to prep your body to receive the benefits of intermittent fasting include:

- Stay hydrated. On average, adults need to drink about 8 glasses of water daily. The human body is made up of about 70% water and needs water to ensure life-sustaining processes are maintained. The process of autophagy needs water to operate the right way as well.
- Get enough sleep every night. Adult needs to get between 7 and 9 hours of sleep nightly for the best health. The body uses this time to repair itself and you should definitely catch the z's you need before starting s fast session.
- Practice stress management. When you are stressed, the body releases stress hormones such as cortisol. These hormones help you in dangerous situations and stress is even a good thing when it is experienced once

in a while. However, chronic stress wears the body down and leads to poor mental and physical health. It also makes it difficult for the processes initiated by intermittent fasting to go smoothly.

You are probably cognizant of the fact that different people can use the same methods to lose weight and get very different results. This is commonly a result of the genes you inherit from your family. Genes are not the only thing playing a role, though. Everyone burns some calories even when they are not exercising, but the rate at which the calories burn depends on your DNA, the current state of your anatomy, and your health history.

It might help you lose weight and maintain healthy weight by keeping track of your calories, but, perhaps even more important, is keeping track of where your calories are coming from. For example, are they coming from nutrient-rich sources, or from calorie-rich, nutrient-poor sources? One of them will help you lose weight, and the other will do the opposite.

How many calories you take in is also important. Logically, you will, of course, lose more weight the fewer calories you consume, but that is not a good thing if you don't eat enough. A woman eating fewer than 900 calories will harm her body more than help it. Intermittent fasting is not about staving yourself or depriving yourself of the calories that you need to stay alive and healthy.

As the saying goes, "slow and steady wins the race." So, you should limit your calories at a steady, reasonable amount. Simply consuming as few calories as possible will not help you in the long run even though many women have been tempted into this practice in an effort to drop several pounds quickly. This is not a safe practice though, and I strongly urge you not to do this. Instead, speak with your doctor about how many calories you can safely reduce in your daily consumption without running into any health risks. This number depends on your height, current weight, age, and level of activity.

Women often ask the question of why are men better able to lose weight than women. The answer is complicated and not just answered as a gift being bestowed on men by the gods. There are several factors involved when it comes to weight loss and the sexes.

One of the biggest contributing factors include the distribution of body fat. Women tend to have a greater share of fat on their bodies compared to muscle, while men tend to have more muscle compared to fat. Since muscle burns more calories than fat, this means that men typically burn fat more easily than women.

The process of digestion provides nutrients to muscles. Men have more muscle on average, so when they digest food, more of their calories go to support their muscle. Women, on the other hand, don't have as much muscle to support, so less of their calorie consumption goes to muscle support. Instead, it is more likely to be stored as fat.

The type of foods consumed also plays a part in the differences in how men and women lose weight. Scientific research compared this. One experiment showed that one group of women tried to lose weight by avoiding unhealthy food, while the other group tried to lose weight by lowering their consumption of calories overall by eating smaller portions. The end result was that the group of women eating fewer calories overall had lower BMIs (body mass indices), by the end of the study.

The same experiment was done on men and suggested that while limiting calories consumed overall could be a better option for women, the kinds of foods consumed may be more important to focus on for men.

Women should put foods in their bodies that contain the nutrients they need and exercise, but when your main goal is losing weight, the likely focus may be on the number of calories consumed. As long as you keep this number at a safe level, you are likely to optimize your success with IF and autophagy. However, all bodies are different so you need you experiment with the two dieting methods to find the one more effective for your weight loss journey.

Another advantage of practicing intermittent fasting is that it allows for consuming fewer calories. When you don't eat at all during a certain window of the day, this reduces the total number of calories you consume per day. That benefit is only one positive effect of intermittent fasting, although it is a terrific benefit. The other benefit that contributes toward weight loss comes from the autophagy process triggered by intermittent fasting. We will have a lot to learn about this process in the upcoming chapters.

But first, let's consider another challenge that women face when it comes to weight loss – the menstrual cycle. Being on your period doesn't make your weight go up or down by a significant permanent amount, but it can influence your weight in indirect ways. For example, you may have more of an appetite for sugary and salty food when you have PMS (premenstrual syndrome). Obviously, eating more foods like these can have quite an effect on your weight, even though your cycle doesn't affect your mass directly. The higher levels of salt in your body can even make your system soak up more water instead of disposing of it, giving you more water weight. This makes losing weight especially troublesome as a Western woman, where sugary and salty foods are widespread and cheap. Your best bet for resisting these temptations is not buying them in the first place. Fill your pantry and fridge with nutrient-rich foods, and don't put the sugary and salty foods there, to begin with.

The same way your period can indirectly affect your weight, your weight can affect your period as well. Although your end goal is to slim down, losing weight or gaining weight in a short span of time can have consequences for your menstrual cycle, as your period may not come on time or may not come at all. Many women with weight problems like obesity have this issue. On the other hand, if your period is coming on schedule on a regular basis, this is a good indicator of good overall health. Accomplishing your goal weight will help make your period come at a regular schedule.

Trying to lose weight can also become a challenge after menopause. On average, menopausal women put on 5 pounds. Menopausal women experience a drop in estrogen levels. Estrogen helps regulate weight, so the fact that estrogen levels are lower may be part of the reason it is harder to lose weight or maintain it.

But we can't blame likely weight gain in that stage of a woman's life solely on menopause. Oftentimes, gaining mass at this stage in life can be due to a slowed metabolism that comes with age in general, eating too many unhealthy foods and not enough healthy ones, and not getting enough exercise.

Women also lose significant muscle mass with age. With less muscle mass comes fewer calorie use by the body. These calories are therefore converted to fat.

All of these facts about losing weight related to menopause cement the fact that all women need to keep an active lifestyle and eat healthful foods.

If you are a woman over the age of 50, it is also recommended that you don't eat as many calories that you used to when you were younger. There are two main reasons for this. First, women don't need as many calories as men because of lower muscle mass, more fat, and being smaller in size in general. Second, women over 50 tend to expend less energy than they used to, so they don't need as many calories in the first place.

If you fall into the demographic of women over 50, you should speak with your doctor about how many calories you can safely limit your diet to lose weight. Their answer may surprise you because women generally don't need as many calories when they are older.

Intermittent Fasting as the Safe and Healthy Alternative to Weight Loss

When women try to slim down, they have many options with which to approach the situation. There are fad new diets, weight loss pills and creams, extreme exercise regimens and more. Unfortunately, many of these alternative will only help you lose weight temporarily if they do work. Most women can sustain these measures in their daily life and so, put the weight back on the moment they get back into their normal routine. Sometimes, they put on even more than their lost. Not only that, but they may have to deal with negative health consequences of using these, many times, unethical means of losing weight.

It is astonishing how many doctors now recommend weight-loss prescriptions to menopausal women. Usually, they will only do this if you have a BMI over 30 (if you are obese), if you are overweight and if you are suffering from other health conditions like hypertension or high cholesterol. It is sad to say but many doctors do not have the health of their patients as their primary interest. Rather, their primary interest is their bottom line.

The responsibility is on you to find good health care and a doctor that has your beast interest at heart. A good doctor will make sure that regular exercise and dieting are part of your regular routine before prescribing you medicine. Prescriptions will only be given to you if you do not see significant results from regular exercise and dieting. While it is understandable to want to avoid the health risks of being overweight or obese, the side effects that accompany these medicines often outweigh the benefits. They include migraines, coughing, tiredness, constipation, and even dissociation.

Again, it makes complete sense that a doctor might prescribe these medications to women so they can lose mass and can be at lower risk for diseases related to weight if the case is extreme. But it is not necessary for you to take these measures and accept these side effects if there are safer alternatives and your case is not extreme. A safer alternative is intermittent fasting.

Intermittent fasting does not have extreme side effects as long as it is practiced safely is an effort to see weight loss. Much like taking a pill, IF doesn't require much change in your daily life. It only requires that you *don't* do something during a small window of your day: eat.

Many modern women are choosing this method over medication because of the many benefits. You can join them today. These upcoming chapters equip you with all the information you need to do IF successfully so you can enjoy its positive effects on your body and health.

Chapter 2 - What is Intermittent Fasting?

"The best of all medicines is resting and fasting."- Benjamin Franklin

Fasting has become a hot topic as of late. The buzz around intermittent fasting, in particular, opened a door for many women who wanted to lose weight but were worried about the heavy commitment of a day-long, water-only fasting. But the part-time nature of intermittent fasting sets it apart from other types of fasting.

When you do an intermittent fast, you are going back and forth in a regular cycle between fasting and eating normally. There is even flexibility within the intermittent fasting process as there are different types of intermittent fasting. I will cover all types of it in this book, and you can decide which best suits your stage in life and goals.

Many women have seen real change happen in their health, thanks to IF. You could join them by following the various tips contained here. The first task we have to complete is giving you a broad overview of:

- What the benefits of intermittent fasting are
- What the science says about intermittent fasting
- What different kinds of intermittent fasting exist
- What foods you should eat as an intermittent faster

Let's start with health benefits. Women who fast intermittently have more energy, burn more fat and lower their chances of getting diabetes or heart disease. Researchers find that IF practitioners have higher success rates than people who do extended, interrupted fasts, and people who use exercise as their chief method to lose weight. Further, they suggest the success of IF is because it is woven seamlessly into the participants' lives. Intermittent fasters do not have to change multiple aspects of their normal routines.

Furthermore, it eliminates the perfectionism that sometimes ruins other weight loss techniques. It doesn't ask that you constantly pay attention to the exact number of calories you consume, and it doesn't punish you harshly for falling out of it for one day.

We will learn more about the science underlying IF later on but suffice to say that you can earn the positive health effects of autophagy without doing extended fasts. The experiments studying people doing IF consistently demonstrate that they see good results from only doing it, without doing more demanding fasts such as extended water fasting.

In the last chapter, we talked about the study showing that women have more success in losing weight by reducing caloric intake compared to when they pay close attention to what they are eating. This is precisely what IF entails. Nutrition is still important, which is why we still have a chapter on it, but regardless of what you eat, you will still likely see some amount of positive change from IF.

I hope that I have at least made you curious about getting these results from IF in your own life — and to do that, you will need to find a way to implement IF in a way that works for you. It's time to answer the question directly... In the simplest terms, what do I have to do to start intermittent fasting today? What is required of me to start seeing these effects on my health?

Do not rush headfirst with your eagerness. Finishing reading to the end of this book first. Then, armed with thorough knowledge, you can start. However, the first thing you need to do is determine the number of hours you will be fasting for.

Let's say your answer is 6 hours. Most beginners start their intermittent fast journey after lunch and break it for dinner. Keep in mind that you will have to eat lunch relatively early so that you do not have dinner too late. If you have dinner too late, your system will take hours to start up autophagy while you sleep. This is because you will still be digesting food as digestion occurs at a slower speed while you sleep. It is as easy as that to start intermittent fasting.

Of course, practice may be harder than theory for some people. I will never tell you that intermittent fasting takes no willpower and resistance on your end. Compared to other potential options, though, it is extremely straightforward especially when you motivate yourself to stick with the process.

You can keep yourself motivate by educating yourself more about the science behind the effectiveness of intermittent fasting and autophagy. You might get inspired when you realize all the delicious foods you can eat when you intermittent fast to make autophagy even stronger. There are many sources of inspiration. You just need to find the one that is perfect for you.

Intermittent Fasting: Looking at its Effects on Health More Closely

Intermittent fasting helps you slim down using short-term and long-term strategies by shortening the supply of calories to your system. This means that you accumulate less fat in the short term and detoxify your cells in the long term through the process of autophagy. The short-term strategy is what tends to draw women in, but the long-term strategy is what makes IF great for your body overall.

This is not the same kind of detox that you may be sick of hearing about online. The autophagy triggered by IF is a detox that has always existed in biology and can be jump-started naturally by fasting. While a detox like "juicing" will claim to clean out your system, supporters of juice diets have no sound data to back up this assertion. Meanwhile, the process of autophagy has been studied by scientists and nutritionists for decades now. It is proven that autophagy supports weight loss and it does so without hurting the body the way that other methods. Not only does it not hurt the body, but it has long-term positive consequences like less inflammation and lower cholesterol.

Every organism on the planet goes through autophagy, so you are not even putting your body through anything strange to get these effects on your health. Even if you had never heard of the word 'autophagy' before, it still occurs in your body. By learning how to trigger it through intermittent fasting, you are simply learning how to optimize the process for your benefit. This procedure doesn't involve the use of any strange medicines or foods either even though your diet does affect how powerful autophagy occurs.

Let's go into more detail on the short-term effects of IF. The practice enhances the health of your skin. The first layer of skin that you have is called the epidermis. You see your epidermis every day because this is the visible part of your skin. There are layers of skin below it, but you don't see those layers unless you suffer an injury.

Both parts of the word "autophagy" are of Greek origin. "Auto" has the meaning "self" and "phagy" has the meaning "eat." Put the two together, and you get the fundamental concept of autophagy. Therefore, your cells "eat themselves" when they are under acute stress. Your cells need energy constantly—even when you are sleeping. They will take it from whatever source they can find. Even when you are not putting food into your body, such as when you are fasting, your cells find ways of getting energy. When in this state of stress, their main sources of energy are the following:

- Cell organelles that stopped working
- Proteins that are no longer being used
- Toxins that came from outside your body

The process of autophagy means that skin cells gain energy is this way and therefore purge themselves of inactive organelles and proteins and toxins. The autophagy results in skin that isn't filled with cellular waste. The skin will look younger because of its resulting newfound elasticity and glow.

The cleaning out of cellular waste isn't the only reason your skin looks and feels better. It's also because there will be an increase in the collagen protein in your skin. Collagen is a protein that your skin cells. It acts as an anchor for skin cells to keep them taut and elastic. Collagen production decreases as we age, hence why we lose the elasticity in our skin as we get older. Autophagy is a game changer that reverses this decline.

Autophagy triggers the manufacture of new cells by building them from scratch using the raw materials obtained from consuming cellular waste or by rejuvenating existing cells with new organelles constructed with raw materials obtained from consuming cellular waste.

The best part is that the improved health of your skin is only the beginning of your improved health when intermittent fasting.

The main reason most people start IF is to lose weight. With weight loss typically comes more healthy skin. Another point relating to skin health and weight loss is that if you lose weight too quickly, you are likely to end up with loose skin. This is not a worry with intermittent fasting as weight loss occurs in a controlled way that allows skin to keep its elasticity. By losing weight through intermittent fasting, you cut down on calories and trigger autophagy at the same time. Thus, poorly performing cells are broken down and replaced with new, young cells. At the least, organelles are replaced with new ones. That's why people who lose weight through intermittent fasting are proven to deal with far fewer issues with loose skin. Not only do they have less loose skin to deal with in the beginning, but they are better able to manage what loose skin they might develop because of the better health of their skin.

Another widespread benefit of the process of autophagy is the intermittent faster having more energy. This is because autophagy makes your cells more efficient and more efficient cells means more energy for you.

As you get older, your cells are less effective than they used to be. They are littered with cellular waste and their cell organs (organelles) are damaged and ineffective and inefficient. Autophagy is the remedy to this problem. It disposes of organelles that aren't performing optimally and of cellular waste and misfolded proteins that are taking up space in your cells without doing anything useful. When all of your cells go through it regularly and take care of these issues, you have more energy because your cells make up all of you, and that makes your system more efficient with energy overall.

Increased energy and improved skin health are not the only positive consequences of autophagy. Autophagy can help fight against several health conditions and sicknesses because of its actions in cells. It is useful in preventing some diseases too. Some of these health conditions and sicknesses include:

- Cancer and tumors

- Alzheimer's disease
- Parkinson's disease
- Huntington's disease
- Heart disease
- Autoimmune failure
- Diabetes

Furthermore, this mechanism has been proven to be incredibly effective for matters of the brain and improving brain health. The process plays a huge role in cleaning out the build ups of proteins in your neurons in the brain. This build up leads to clogging and brain dysfunction.

As autophagy occurs in the brain, a special organelle called the autophagosome binds with your lysosome (your cell's stomach in essence) to break down the cellular waste. However, what causes the protein build-ups is the abnormally strong bond that the autophagosome can form with the lysosome. This strong bond between the autophagosome and the lysosome causes what is called a "clogging effect." The clogging effect makes your proteins build up in your neurons, leading to neurodegeneration.

If you want to prevent these neurodegenerative diseases like Parkinson's disease, you have to trigger autophagy as often as possible so your cells clean out your proteins. You might think this sounds counterintuitive since these build-ups happen in the first place because of autophagy occurring and leading to the autophagosome binding too tightly with the lysosome. However, this abnormal binding is only an issue when autophagy is occurring at a maintenance level. Maintenance mod describes autophagy when it is happening at a low level as it does normally. You see, this is always happening in your body somewhere, but that does not mean it is happening at a significant level.

When autophagy only happens in maintenance mode, you do not trigger the advanced process to clean out the resulting protein build-up. All you have to do to clear out this protein build-up is do intermittent fasting. This triggers a heightened level of autophagy , and prevents the protein build-up that can cause neurodegeneration.

While this won't apply to every woman's situation, there has also been testing on the effects of autophagy on people going through chemotherapy for cancer. The researchers looked at a group going through therapy without intermittent fasting and a group who did IF during the chemotherapy.

The group that fasted while going through chemotherapy had significantly lower amounts of dead white blood cells in their systems. If you don't know already, chemotherapy has some negative side effects of killing good cells like white blood cells in addition to killing cancerous cells.

White blood cells do the very important job of protecting the body from infections and disease when they are alive, but like every other cell, they become toxic when they die. Unfortunately, chemotherapy tends to kill a lot of white blood cells in the process of killing cancer cells.

Intermittent fasting can help decrease the number of white blood cells destroyed in chemotherapy. The patients who fasted during chemotherapy had significantly less dead white blood cells creating toxins in their bodies because intermittent fasting got rid of them. IF led their bodies to seek nutrients from inside the body. There were a lot of dead white blood cells in their body, so autophagy took care of those. As a result, they did not have all these dead cells polluting their bodies.

Another study looked at women who were former breast cancer patients who did a fast lasting 12 hours daily. These women did not see their cancer return as often as women who did not fast. This means that not only does intermittent fasting have implications for lessening the side effects of common cancer treatment like chemotherapy, but it can even lower the chances that cancer will come back once it is defeated. Also, it has even been shown that mice who were bred in a lab who went through autophagy triggered through fasting had lower rates of cancer than rats who did not fast. The ones who did not trigger it had higher rates of cancer.

As far as the long-term benefits of autophagy go, it has even been shown to lower the amount of inflammation in your body. Inflammation is a healthy part of a well-functioning immune system but when inflammation persists this can do more harm than good. Autophagy help keep inflammation at a healthy level. When you have less inflammation in your body, DNA in cells is far less likely to be damaged. Damaged DNA and high inflammation are big risk factors for disease developments like cancer, so these are highly important long-term effects.

People often underestimate the importance of their gut healthy but your digestive health is surprisingly to your long-term health outcomes, and autophagy can help keep system healthy as well. If you are not able to get nutrients with a healthy gut, none of the other systems in your body are able to work the way they should.

Your digestive system is constantly working. Its parts never stop, not even when you sleep. Intermittent fasting allows your digestive system to have a smaller work load though and this allows it time to and do repairs as necessary. Autophagy gives the tissues in your digestive system the opportunity to clear out cellular waste to make the system more efficient on the cellular level.

We would be remiss to forget about your autoimmune system in the context of autophagy. Your autoimmune system is the one that keeps you safe from the attack of infections and disease. It helps fight cancer cells before they can grow to the size of a tumor. But your immune response isn't limited to it reaction to the presence of cancer. Your autoimmune system keeps all foreign entities at bay and from harming your body.

Doctors say that preventive medicine is the most important kind of medicine, and your autoimmune system is the main player in your body's natural disease preventive mechanism. Intermittent fasting helps keep this vital system healthy and operating at maximum while preventing age-related disease.

However, you can't expect to get these results by practicing intermittent fasting every once in a while. If you eat poorly, consume a lot of alcohol, smoke, get little sleep, or have any number of habits that are bad for your health, you can't expect to do IF and have it repair all the damage you do to your body from these habits. Successfully triggering autophagy with intermittent fasting to gain the benefits discussed requires that you are healthy. You know yourself. That means that you know the bad habits that you practice that are detrimental to the health of your body. To make intermittent fasting and the process of autophagy work for you, you need to first make the lifestyle shift that encompasses healthy habits.

A Closer Look at Autophagy
Autophagy is the natural way your body disposes of toxic chemicals in your cells. You can't see it happening without a microscope, but your cells have been going through it for your entire life without you even noticing. In just the last twenty years, scientists have learned much about the metabolic process than ever before. They have learned more and more about its implications for fighting against disease, aging and weight loss.

The entire foundation of using intermittent fasting for losing weight and getting healthier is founded on our scientific understanding of autophagy. We know for a fact that it can help us attain better general health and live longer. But is not just modern civilization that has benefited from the process. In fact, our ancestors utilized the process part more that we do. Autophagy was a frequently occurring process back in the days before industrial agriculture because human begin did not expect to have food all the time.

Nowadays, in the industrialized world, most people rarely miss a meal. We always have food around us, but people back in the day did not even have an expectation of eating every single day. Our bodies went through advanced autophagy very regularly because of this, and we can even say that our bodies are more built for not eating every day than they are for constantly eating as we do right now.

Our first encounter with this mechanism in the world of science was thanks to the French scientist named Christian De Duve. He and a group of biologists took note of a bizarre organelle that they had never seen before. They named it the lysosome.

Scientists thought that the lysosome was simply an organelle made for disposing of garbage. If you think about it, this doesn't even make logical sense, because there is not really such thing as disposing of something. You can change the form of something, but not dispose of it. If the lysosome was really an organelle that just kept breaking things down without recycling those parts, then eventually those tiny waste particles would build-up with nowhere to go.

Now we have an explanation for this problem because of autophagy, and this explanation has important takeaways for doctors, biologists, and anyone who cares about their health.

The Japanese scientist Yoshinori Ohsumi was the first scientist to get deeply interested in the lysosome of yeast cells. 2016 was the year he won the Nobel Prize because he was the one who learned that the lysosome was the center of a cellular process called autophagy. His key finding was that our cells never "dispose of" anything. They simply break down cellular waste into raw materials, and then use these materials to build new structures.

Ohsumi has created a new definition of this process. He says that it is the way our cells break down waste materials for the purpose of freeing up space, killing harmful foreign toxins, and creating raw materials that can be used for building new cells. When Ohsumi first started, he was the first scientist to really have any interest in this topic. He started a scientific movement around it when his research uncovered all the implications that autophagy has for our bodies. Not only did Ohsumi uncover much of our modern understanding of autophagy, but he was the one who coined the phrase "cell recycling." Cell recycling is what happens once autophagy is finished.

When your cells have cleaned themselves out, they use these raw materials for constructing things that other cells can use. They can also use these raw materials to create new cells if there is enough.

Now we know that this can be considered the most important process for your cells both individually and collectively. It matters to your cells individually because it keeps them alive. It matters collectively because your cells have to work together to be useful to your body as a whole, and it keeps them working together smoothly when the process keeps them repaired and "cleaned out."

The Ideal Diet for a Woman Doing Intermittent Fasting

Before we dive into the subject of what you eat when you fast, I need to issue a warning to you: there are people selling supplements that they say will trigger autophagy. At the moment, no such supplements exist. That means you need to be wary of claims like these. There are scientists trying to create a medication with this effect, but it has not been made yet.

Eating the right foods in addition to intermittent fasting is your best bet on triggering autophagy safely and healthily. Vitamin D is the first nutritional content that needs to be had for autophagy to occur. And here's the best part! You don't need to eat any food to get that nutrition. All you have to do is go soak up some sun.

Vitamin D is an essential vitamin to a myriad of biological processes that your system goes through, and autophagy is one of them. Supplement the amount of vitamin D that you get from going out in the sun by eating these foods:

- Fortified foods like breakfast cereals
- Liver
- A moderate amount of red meat
- Oily fish like sardines, salmon and mackerel
- Egg yolks

Ginger is a food that has nutritional value that triggers autophagy. It contains a chemical called 6-shogaol, which actually slows the growth of cells in your lungs. It probably seems counterproductive to ingest something that stops your cells from growing when you are trying to prevent cancer or some other lung disease. However, ginger is an excellent complement to autophagy because this chemical suppresses cell growth. 6-shogaol suppresses all cell growth, meaning that even cancer cells will not be able to grow as well when you add this chemical into your system.

Omega-3 fats are probably something that you have heard of before. They are considered a "healthy fat," a kind of fat that your body needs. People who get plenty of these healthy fats into their bodies have been shown to have more advanced autophagy than people who do not. So, it is greatly aided by unsaturated fats like Omega-3 fats.

With that in mind, you should know that with Omega-3 fats and all of the nutrients we mention, you need to make a real effort to get them from your regular diet rather than from supplements. Get the real thing where possible. Great natural sources of Omega-3 fats include:

- Oily fish like sardines, salmon, tuna, anchovies and mackerel
- Plant oils like soybean oil, flaxseed oils and canola oils
- Seeds and nuts like chia seeds, walnuts and flaxseeds.

Another point against getting your Omega-3 fats from a supermarket is that grocery stores these supplements are known to get their meats from factory farms. Meat coming from factory farms does not have Omega-3 fats because of what factory farms feed their cattle. Instead of eating grass or other natural foods, they consume a lot of chemicals. Instead of indirectly getting the Omega-3 fats from grass through your meat, you are indirectly getting whatever chemical foods these factory farms give to their animals.

It goes without saying that you need to eat plenty of vegetables when you are doing intermittent fasting, too. It is a simple fact that a lot of people don't like vegetables at all, but thankfully there are ways of getting around this. One of them is putting your vegetables in a blender together with some fruit to create smoothies. If you get your vegetables this way, you should remember not to add too much fruit into the blender. While fruits are good for us, they have a lot of natural sugar in them, which is still bad for us in large quantities, just like artificial sugars.

The next thing you should consider consuming to help the autophagy processes is green tea. The chemical in green tea that you are really looking for is called AMPK. This is an enzyme that boosts the effectiveness of autophagy. Turmeric consumption works in a similar way to digesting green tea as it relates to triggering autophagy.

Reishi mushrooms are also great at triggering autophagy. The reishi mushroom is a special case because it can significantly slow the growth of one cell in particular: cancer cells in the colon. The colon is a common place to start seeing cancer, so this food is really something that you should consider adding to your diet. It works by helping the growth of non-cancer cells when cancer cells are growing in the colon. When non-cancer cells are able to grow and flourish in your body alongside cancer cells, this really helps keep cancer at bay and fight it. Each cell does its part in trying to overwhelm the cancer cells. Normally, the cancer cells in the colon will actively try to stop the non-cancer cells from growing, and the chemicals in the reishi mushroom do their part in keeping this from occurring.

Looking at autophagy and intermittent fasting from the perspective of diet can be very inspiring because you can look at them from more than one point of view. You feel as though you are triggering autophagy in every way possible from the simple action of eating certain foods that you know for sure are helpful.

Good practitioners of these two mechanisms will use several methods to make their autophagy as strong as possible. I have done extensive research about what scientists say on these different diets, and I am only recommending foods to you that are proved to work.

If you are still having issues deciding which approach is right for you, looking at the foods you eat might be a good place to start. This book strongly recommends IF since it is known to be the most consistent way of getting more autophagy to happen in your system, but everyone is different, so you might want to think about all of your options.

You also need to think about what not to eat when you are thinking about autophagy. Our number one enemy against it is carbs. Everyone knows about the bad reputation that carbs have, but not enough know exactly why we should lessen how many carbs we put into our bodies. Did you know that the average American gets nearly 60% of their calories every day from carbs? It seems incredible, but it's true. Not only do American women have the issue of eating a lot of calories without a plan to burn them off with exercise, but they are getting many of these calories from a source that is notorious for being converted into fat cells.

Here is the true reason that makes carbs so dangerous, especially for someone who has a plan to do IF. When your gut is holding all of your foods and breaking them down, it has proteins, fats, and carbohydrates. No matter how much fat and protein it has to break down, no matter what other factors are at play, your body will always break down carbs first. Carbs get turned to fat when they are not used up.

Also, carbs are not an efficient energy source as the body burns through them quickly and then demands more carbs to make up for that interruption in the supply of energy. Fats and protein are much more efficient supplies of energy but in the presence of carbs, the body does not use them for energy.

You need to choose a diet that is very low in carbs if you want to succeed in intermittent fasting.

Your new life as a slimmer, healthier, and more youthful woman depends upon you eating fewer carbs. You will be surprised how many times a day carbs make their way into your diet. This will seriously impair your autophagy. Another way of illustrating this is by looking at how much it reduces it.

We can use an example where you finish eating a meal at 1 pm and then stop eating until 9 pm. This seems like an 8-hour fast. However, it really is a 4-hour fast. This is because when you stop eating at 1 pm, it takes your body 4 hours to digest your food. You aren't done digesting it until 5 pm, and then you start eating again at 9 pm. Thus, your fast was really 4 hours long. Now, let's put carbohydrates into the picture. Let's say the last meal you eat before you start fasting is a bowl filled with pasta at 1 pm, and then you don't eat again until 9 pm. Take a guess at how long of a fast this really was.

The answer is 0 hours. That's right: it takes 8 hours for your body to digest carbs. Even though you stop eating for 8 hours after the bowl of pasta, your stomach is just now finishing digesting the carbs from the pasta at 9 pm, and then you are just putting more food into your body again, stopping autophagy. The latter depends heavily on what you are consuming. It relies on you getting plenty of healthy fats and not eating too many carbs. Practically speaking, most people doing IF to lose weight should reduce their consumption of carbs to be as low as possible.

Now, we need to spend some time talking about fats. It can be confusing because a lot of people are under the impression that fats are bad overall. They don't realize how much their bodies rely on fats to perform basic functions—including autophagy. Not all fats are the same. Because of the chemical composition of different fats, some of them are essential, while some of them should be limited to being eaten as little as possible. The fats in your diet can be the hardest thing for you to control, and the way it works can be hard to understand. They can be some of the best things for your body and some of the worst things for your body. First, we will get into what can make them good when you eat the right ones.

Firstly, your system depends on fats because they are one of its sources of energy. Fats can even store vitamins and minerals. Fats are essential for building membranes around your cells and sheaths around your nerves. On a bigger scale, you have fat for moving your muscles, clotting your blood, and keeping your inflammation at normal levels. Generally, we can say that your saturated fats are bad for you, and your unsaturated fats are good for you. Trans fats are especially bad for you, but you don't have to think about that too much, because now they are banned in most places.

Trans fats are a great demonstration of what can make your fats bad. These kinds of fats only come into being because of the industrial, artificial processes that create and preserve food these days. They have no use in your body and can only harm you.

Then you have saturated fats. Doctors say that you should be keeping your level of saturated fats to less than 10% of all your calories. If at all possible, don't eat saturated fats when you have them as an option.

Meanwhile, doctors want us to get about 30% of our calories from good fats. To a lot of people, this seems like a lot of fats for doctors to recommend to us! It goes to show you how different kinds of fats have such different effects on our bodies.

We have plenty more to discuss in the chapter coming later about what foods to eat when doing IF, but this should give you a good preview of what to expect later. Now you can read about what different options you have for methods of intermittent fasting.

The Keto Diet and Intermittent Fasting

We have discussed the benefits of diminishing the number of carbs you consume on a daily basis as an intermittent faster.

That can be difficult to do on the average diet but there is one diet whose main selling point is that it is based on eating as few carbs as possible.

It is called the ketogenic diet. It is also called the keto diet for short. You may have already heard about the keto diet since it is trending in popularity right now. However, this diet did not just spring out of nowhere. It has been around for over a century. Although the initial invention of this diet was to help patients suffering from epilepsy control their symptoms, it was found that this diet was particularly helpful in gaining many other health benefits and one of the most interesting was weight loss.

This diet does not just promote low-carb eating but also high fat and moderate protein intake. The standard keto diet has an eating ratio that looks like this:

- 5% carbohydrates
- 20% protein
- 75% fat

The keto diet is used by millions of people worldwide to gain benefits like:

- Better weight management
- Decreased risk of developing some cancers and in the treatment of some cancers and tumor
- Decreased risk of developing type 2 diabetes due to fat loss and increased insulin sensitivity
- Decreased incidence of acne breakouts
- Reduced risk of developing polycystic ovarian syndrome.
- Decreased risk of developing cardiovascular diseases

A diet that is high in fat might seem to be contrary to losing weight at first glance but the validity of this diet cannot be beaten on closer inspection. The diet works because it uses specific fats and does not practice just eating fats indiscriminately. So not, just going out and eating a pound of butter is not what this diet is about. Rather, it is about making smart, healthy choices about fat intake while limiting the consumption of carbs.

The keto diet is so effective in so many health improvements because it makes the body turn away from using carbs as its main energy source and instead burns fats as the main energy source. When the body is short on carbs it kick starts a process known as ketosis. This is also a metabolic process just like the burning of carbs for energy. Ketosis is initiated during times of pregnancy, starvation, practicing the keto diet and, of course, fasting.

The name ketosis comes from the metabolic products produced by the process. These metabolic products are called the ketones and they are fat-derived molecules of energy that are produced in the liver and then flow through the bloodstream. There are three types of ketones. They are:

- Acetoacetate
- Beta-hydroxybutyrate
- Acetone

Ketones are not just magical produced only during times when the body undergoes ketosis. They are always present in some concentration in your blood but when the body undergoes ketosis, their concentration magnifies dramatically so that the body is forced to use them as an energy source as they outnumber the presence of carbohydrates.

This diet promotes weight loss because fat molecules are burnt to form ketones, which leads to a natural way of slimming down. Practitioners of the keto diet also slim down because they typically feel fuller and more satisfied after they eat meals. After all, it is higher in fat and proteins, which are not used as quickly as carbohydrates. Due to feeling fuller and more satisfied, a person is also less likely to overeat and the appetite is reduced as well. This leads to a lessened likelihood of reaching for snacks, which are abundant in the carbohydrate variety.

It might be difficult to tell if a person is relying on ketosis to get their body fueled but there are a few signs that you will notice if you know what to look out for. The typical signs that a body is relying on ketosis for energy include:

- Decreased appetite due to the suppression of hormones that make you feel hungry.
- Initial feelings of fatigue due to the body adjusting to this new energy supply. These feelings typically go away in a few days as the body learns to adapt to this new supply of cleaner energy.
- Experiencing initial feelings of constipation and diarrhea due to the body adjusting to this new diet. These digestive issues are typically a sign of transition and normally go away in a few days so this is no cause for you to worry.
- Increased mental focus and concentration because the brain works more efficiently on energy supplied this way.
- Fruity smelling breath. This is normally a symptom that some people like but if you do not, all you have to do is brush your teeth or use sugar-free gum to get rid of the smell.

For this process to be initiated, the person must consume less than 50g of carbs a day. That means taking out high-sugar foods and the foods we discussed above from the diet. This means that other high-carb options must be eliminated as well.

Foods that must not be consumed on the keto diet include:

- Baked goods such as cookies
- Most bread like white and wheat bread
- Grains like rice and pasta
- Sweeteners like honey and maple syrup
- Root vegetables like carrots and potatoes
- Beans and legumes
- Condiments and sauces like ketchup and BBQ sauce, as they normally contain high amounts of sugar and unhealthy fats
- Alcohol
- All fruits except for a few berries

Foods that contain unhealthy fat called trans fats need to be avoided as well. Remember that you need to be highly partial when it comes to picking the fats that you consumed with this diet. Trans fats come from processed foods that have been produced with partially hydrogenated oil. It is imperative that you read food labels when you grocery shop. Any items that list these names in their ingredient list needs to be left on the grocery shelf.

Foods that are safe for eating on the keto diet are:

- Means like chicken and beef
- Fatty fish like tuna and sardines
- Shellfish and other seafood
- Full-fat dairy
- Avocados
- Nuts and seeds
- Cruciferous vegetables like broccoli and cauliflower

- Other veggies that are low in carb content like peppers and onions
- Dark chocolate
- Condiments that are low in sugar content like salt, pepper and mustard
- Berries like blackberries, blueberries and raspberries because they are low in sugar by relatively high in healthy fat content
- Sweeteners like stevia and erythritol but only when used in moderation
- Healthy oils like virgin olive oil, avocado oil and sunflower oil. They contain good-for-you fats like monounsaturated and polyunsaturated fats.

The keto diet also helps turn on autophagy because it involves depriving your body of the carbs that it would normally consume for energy. To understand how ketosis kick starts autophagy, we need to take a closer look into how the process of ketosis is activated and how it is propagated until energy is produced so that your organs are able to utilize it.

Before ketosis ever happens the process of gluconeogenesis occurs. Because the body is already running low on a supply of carbohydrates to produce the energy it needs, it will look for non carbohydrate components to produce this energy. The first thing that it typically looks for is amino acids, which are the individual components that make up proteins, to produce this energy. Ketones get produced in a little bit of a higher quantity but still lower than necessary to kick start ketosis. The supply will quickly run out and then ketosis will occur as these non-carbohydrate components run low.

When ketosis is finally initiated in full force, the liver produces ketones out of fat cells that have been broken down in the process known as ketogenesis. The first ketone to be produced is acetoacetate. This ketone is then converted into beta-hydroxybutyrate and acetone. As your body adjusts to this new energy supply, the ketone which is the most frequently found in your bloodstream and organs as an energy supply is beta-hydroxybutyrate. When your body is running in full ketosis mode, more than 50% of its energy is derived from the process while the brain derives up to 70% of its energy needs from this process.

When your body is in the process of gluconeogenesis and its supply of carbohydrates is running out, this initiates autophagy because your cells are desperately seeking an energy source.

Therefore, in conjunction with being an intermittent faster, it might be the best prerogative for you to adopt the ketogenic diet as part of your daily lifestyle. While it can seem like an abrupt change from the norm, once you get into the swing of things it will come naturally to live by this diet. The added energy and weight loss, among the many other benefits, more than make it worth it to at least consider practicing this diet.

Different Methods of Fasting

As we continue to discuss the methods of intermittent fasting you will surely find at least one that suits your needs. But intermittent fasting is not the only type of fasting.

I will start by telling you that IF is by far the most popular way to fast overall. Outside of it, the only other legitimate option is called extended water fasting. Extended water fasting, usually just called water fasting, is when you only consume water for a period of time, usually lasting 24 hours or longer. We will get into it a little bit in this book, but there are many reasons that we will mostly stick to intermittent fasting.

I say that the non-intermittent fasts outside of water fasting are not legitimate simply because there is no research supporting their claims the way there is for both of them. We will start by talking about what other fasts you may hear about, and I will tell you why you can forget about them entirely, because either they won't work to help you lose weight, they are bad for your body, or oftentimes, both. The most dangerous one is called dry fasting. Dry fasting caries the same concepts as water fasting, but you don't even consume water. It is hard to say why this idea even exists because there is no reason to believe that it would be more effective in helping you lose weight than water fasting. Sure, you will lose water weight for a temporary span of time, but then you will go back to drinking water and gain it all back again. It does not even keep the water weight off of you.

But all of that is beside the point; you don't want to lose water weight. Hydration is one of the most important things to be mindful of when caring for your body, and when it gets too low, that is bad for you in general—not to mention bad for your autophagy. I said to watch your diet, exercise, fasting, and sleep when you want to trigger it, but you have to watch your water consumption, too. Not having any water for your cells dries them out and prevents them from working the way that they should.

Once you get a grip on the intermittent fasting stuff, you might want to dip your toes into water fasting. The best way to do this is by participating in the 24-hour fast.

When you do a true, traditional fast, you don't eat at all for at least a day. This is the essence of the water fast, too, but extended this process can last for multiple days. With the 24-hour fast, you are only dedicating yourself to fasting for 24 hours.

Next, we have what is known as consecutive day fasting. If fasting for a set number of hours every single day sounds like a commitment that you won't be able to keep up, then fasting for consecutive day fasting will hardly be the right choice for you. Consecutive day fasting involves not eating for at least 2 consecutive days at least once a month. The practitioner can drink fluid during the fast and needs to slowly reintroduce foods after the fast. There are obvious drawbacks to this type of fast such as severe hunger, fatigue, dizziness and insomnia.

When it comes to fasts that you should strictly avoid, we could talk about protein fasting. Protein fasting is when protein is the only thing that you consume. Protein may be an important thing for you to get into your system, but it is definitely not wise to make it the only nutrient you get. In fact, it is best for you to eat a pretty low amount of it. Your body will break down protein before fat, and as a result, your autophagy will be better if you don't eat as much of it. The logic behind this method of fasting simply doesn't hold up, so you shouldn't pay any attention to it.

Chapter 3 - Benefits of Intermittent Fasting

"Fasting from any nourishment, activity, involvement or pursuit—for any season—sets the stage for God to appear. Fasting is not a tool to pry wisdom out of God's hands or to force needed insight about a decision. Fasting is not a tool for gaining discipline or developing piety (whatever that might be). Instead, fasting is the bulimic act of ridding ourselves of our fullness to attune our senses to the mysteries that swirl in and around us."—Dan B. Allender, PhD

There is no longer a debate on this point: intermittent fasting has many significant and positive consequences for your health. People who have it as part of their routine say their minds feel clearer, and they are capable of more productive work because their bodies have more energy. They report an increase in muscle mass and a decrease in body fat. Insulin goes down, your skin gets a glow and is more elastic, and your heart is healthier. And all these benefits came from, when you really break it down, simply skipping a meal or two a day.

We just summarized many of these positive health effects in the previous chapter, but in this chapter, let's take the opportunity to provide you with even more knowledge about how intermittent fasting will improve your body's health.

Autophagy: Nature's Detoxifier

Now that you have learned the science underlying the benefits of autophagy, we can dive deeper into the cleansing side of it. The science behind it is what makes intermittent fasting better than other strategies. It tells us that it is something that all of us should be thinking about—even if we are not trying to lose weight—because it just has that much influence on our bodies.

Even as you read into the third chapter, I can guarantee you that you have not yet scratched the surface of what intermittent fasting, and so autophagy, will do for your body once you find yourself doing it every day. Look at it this way: there is definitely a lot of evidence that kale is a superfood that is very good for you since it is filled with so many vitamins and nutrients that your body needs. That's why everyone says that you should eat it.

Some people take scientific facts, like kale being good for you, and twist them to make it seem like kale is the only food you should be eating. They try to sell you diets based on blending kale and drinking it throughout the day. While it's true that consuming more kale would be good for you, it still doesn't compare to adding kale to your diet to enhance your diet. The same analogy can be applied to intermittent fasting. Yes, it has the potential to work in its own to help you lose weight and gain other benefits but when combined with other good habits like eating healthy, sleeping 8 hours every night and exercising regularly, the benefits are almost certain and far more than you would have hoped by just intermittent fasting alone.

Intermittent fasting trigger autophagy and autophagy is essential to your body. It happens whether you like it or not, and if you never thought about it in your whole life, it would still happen. If your cells didn't go through it, your cells would die, and you would die along with them. This is what makes detoxifying your body with autophagy different from detoxifying your body with something like kale. We are taking something that your body already does and needs and maximizing it to its greatest potential.

No matter how much energy you feel like you are using at any given time, your cells are always using energy. They do not get to sleep and recover from a long day. This is what makes autophagy a central part of a cell's functions. When you fast, and your cells' energy resources are depleted, they still need the energy to keep on going.

So, they find that energy in the nooks and crannies. Your cells eat their own unused proteins, broken organelles, and their autophagosomes start working extra hard to find the toxins that are in various parts of your system. Autophagosomes are parts of the cells slated for autophagy. Your cells are extra motivated to benefit from autophagy when you fast because if they don't, they can't keep doing the things that cells do.

Our cells don't care about their state of cleanliness the way you do. You care about their cleanliness because they work much better when they have cleared out the toxins, and that's where all the positive health effects of autophagy come from. Since your cells don't care themselves, they will let things get very crowded. They will have toxins all over and will simply die when it becomes so much that they can't work properly.

Of course, they will eventually go through some maintenance mode autophagy when you go to sleep. But you are reading this book because you want your cells to go above and beyond what they would normally do… Because that is what is going to get the best health outcomes for you.

We really let our cells make a mess of themselves in the modern-day with all the junk food and fast food that we eat. The sheer amount that we eat also contributes to this pile up of toxins. Once you do your first intermittent fast, you will realize how much we eat every day like it's nothing.

To briefly look at things from a philosophical standpoint, we are always filling ourselves with stuff, and we don't give ourselves a chance to empty ourselves out. Autophagy comes in for that last part. Our bodies are not anywhere equipped to deal with all the junk we stuff into our bodies these days, so we have to think about our cells proactively and make sure they use this process to keep things running efficiently.

We all know the artificial chemicals that inevitably end up in our bodies in today's society. If we don't deliberatively take care of it by doing intermittent fasting, some of these may end up having negative long-term consequences on our health. I don't advocate for being paranoid about what chemicals are in our foods, but it is a simple fact that our foods are filled with them, and we can't be certain that all of them are fine for us. It may not be possible for us to get rid of these chemicals in our lives completely, but we can get rid of the ones that do end up in our bodies using the natural cleansing process of autophagy.

Not only will you get rid of these toxins for the sake of your general health, but having a clean system leaves you feeling great, too. You can really feel the difference subjectively. We talk a lot about the physical health side of things in this book, but we can't ignore the emotional element. Having the peace of mind that your body is consistently getting rid of toxins can be relieving in trying times. Using IF is not only about optimizing your physical health as much as possible, but your psychological health as well.

When the detox is a big part of what you want autophagy to do for you, you may be motivated to make it as potent as possible by using a variety of triggering methods. IF should be your main method of triggering autophagy since it is the easiest, and therefore, the most reliable. But once you start feeling the difference in your skin and under it—once the work your cells are doing is a sensation you detect it throughout your biological systems—there is a good chance you will fall in love with it and want more.

You can combine intermittent fasting with other techniques to make your detox as powerful as possible. If you have a sauna in your community that you can visit, it could be helpful. Saunas do so much good for your body, as they will make your heart rate go remain steady, improve the circulation of your blood, and do a detox on your body directly through your skin. Saunas do this because they put your cells into a state of stress. If you recall, this state of stress is the thing that puts your cells into autophagy. Intermittent fasting is the best way to trigger the state of stress on a daily, reliable basis, but saunas will help, too, heightening your natural detox.

Even if you don't have a sauna, you can get some of the benefits of taking a hot shower, as the steam will seep into your skin and do some of the detoxification that a sauna would do. Thus, your cells will get some of the state of stress that would come from a sauna. None of this is to say that a sauna or hot shower should replace intermittent fasting—they shouldn't, because they don't allow advance autophagy like intermittent fasting does. However, if you use these methods alongside intermittent fasting, the autophagy you get will increase.

Autophagy and Your Skin

Now that you know more about the science of it, we can go deeper into the health benefits that IF will confer to your skin.

First of all, you should know how important hydration is to your skin. You may be going through autophagy 12 hours a day and still not see improvement in your skin if you are not properly hydrated. Most people do not get enough water every day. Be sure you are drinking 8 glasses a day, at the very least. This is truthfully the best thing you can do for your skin.

Earlier, you learned how intermittent fasting and autophagy detoxify your system. Well, this means that your pores are cleared out, too. No one wants to keep their pores clogged. It leads to greasy-looking skin and acne development. If you drink plenty of water and keep up your habit of intermittent fasting, you won't have to worry about clogged pores in your skin for much longer unless there is some underlying problem preventing that.

The way that IF improves your skin works in two ways. For one, it unclogs these pores, since autophagy breaks down the toxins that clog them up. It also makes your skin cells healthier overall. This results in the long-term and more desired effect of more elastic and more youthful skin.

To you keep your skin healthy with autophagy, your true goal is to increase the amount of collagen that your skin cells produce. We went into this topic in the last chapter, but now we have the space to go into more detail.

Not all of your skin cells produce the collagen protein. Some of them do. These skin cells are called fibroblasts. Fibroblasts are specialized cells made to produce the protein we have been talking about known as collagen.

You can't go wrong with collagen—the more you have of it, the healthier and more elastic your skin is. Unfortunately though, even by the time we turn 18 years of age, our fibroblasts start producing less collagen. Our skin starts getting less stretchy as a result. If you want more collagen, you have to take care of your cells by drinking lots of water and doing IF to trigger autophagy. Our fibroblasts stop making as much collagen because they get clogged up with toxins, just like our pores. These cells are not as efficient since they are so crowded out by toxins. The unused proteins, organelles, and other toxins start to add up and create real problems for your fibroblast's functioning.

This is what we mean when we say that autophagy helps your skin in two ways because one triggers the other to clean out your pores, but this reduction in toxins also ends up making your fibroblasts healthier and more efficient. More efficient cells are able to do their job properly; fibroblasts get better at producing collagen, and your skin gets tighter.

Taking care of your skin is not only a matter of appearance, although there is nothing wrong with wanting to manage your looks too. Your skin is one of your most important organs. Healthier skin protects you against skin cancer, ultraviolet rays, and diseases trying to permeate through your skin cells' membranes.

Your skin cells get replaced a lot. All of them get replaced every month. Autophagy is integral to this non-stop process of renewal in your skin cells. Triggering it with IF will result in these health benefits because you are protecting the continuous cycle of skin cells that you need to protect your body.

To detoxify your body, your skin is the best place to start. It serves as your first line of defense against the toxins that enter your body from the outside.

It is also necessary to get better, healthier skin because it has the capacity to tackle this continual cycle of new cells in your skin. No other method can deal with the constant stream of new skin cells, which is why they tend to fail.

For instance, there are endless skincare products that claim to do what autophagy really does for your skin, but this is impossible since these products can't compete with the way autophagy works deep in the layers of skin to renew old cells and develop new cells.

These skincare products can only penetrate the top of your outermost layer of skin, possibly making it look better. But they are only covering it up the problem without solving the issue that can only be solved through cellular means.

It is unfortunate that so many people waste their time and money on products that don't work, but at least you won't have to. In fact, the improved health and youthfulness of your skin will probably be the first thing you notice as a result of intermittent fasting. Along with weight loss, it is commonly reported as the first noticeable difference.

The desire to lose weight and get better skin often goes together. One reason for this is fear of the so-called "skin curtain." We already discussed this fear briefly, but I want to be sure that you do not let this irrational fear hold you back from making lifestyle changes that are good for your body. Like we said before, loose skin from weight loss has a lot of factors that go into it, such as:

- The speed at which you lose the weight
- How much weight is lost
- Genetics
- Age
- The health of your skin.

Not only can we deal with loose skin to once you have it, but also a lot of these things can be prevented in the first place. We can control them. Let's get into controlling loose skin once we have it.

Probably the biggest reason we shouldn't worry about loose skin from weight loss is that it isn't permanent. Of course, these things always go on a case-by-case basis, but most people who are looking at loose skin after weight loss don't have to accept it into their lives. There are a variety of ways that it can be managed if you have it, and surgery isn't the only option. Working to do without loose skin is a lot like taking care of your skin in general. You want to drink 8 or more glasses of water a day, get adequate exercise, and get the essential nutrients from your diet.

It takes time to tighten up your loose skin, for sure, but this is a much easier problem to deal with than excess fat on your body. It is incredible how many people are reluctant to slim down because of their irrational fear of loose skin. Don't let yourself be one of them. In short, loose skin can be handled once you lose weight. It is not permanent; just like being overweight or obese isn't permanent. Just like those things, you just have to put in the work consistently and be patient as time does its part in tightening up loose skin from weight loss.

You can keep the loose skin from being a problem in the first place, too. Your age and how much weight you need to lose are not things that you can control, but you can control other things such as how much water you drink, how quickly you lose weight, whether you get enough nutrients, and whether you exercise.

Take care of the things you can control, and if you still have some loose skin when the weight is off, keep taking care of your body and keep following your IF routine, so your skin tightens as quickly as possible.

It's true that your skin is the organ that everyone can see, and this is why there is a multi-million-dollar industry to help people improve their skin health. However, the way your skin looks should not be the main thing that you are concerned about. It is just like how people want to lose weight to look better, but losing weight will also decrease their health risks for heart disease and cancer, too. Women, in particular, need to pay close attention to the health of their skin, because sometimes they use so many products on them that they are unsure of the natural state of their skin health.

After you take a shower, inspect your skin, and evaluate how healthy you think it is. Inspecting your skin regularly will get you motivated to keep on your IF regimen. You will see improvements very quickly. Your skin's main purpose is not to look nice, but to protect your body from toxins on the outside. Doing IF will help you protect your skin, empowering it to shield your system from pathogens and microbes. Thankfully, taking care of your skin will also make it look better. It is a win-win situation.

Autophagy and Your Energy
Everyone who intermittently fasts says the same thing: they can do so much more now every day than they used to be able to because they have more energy.

You already know that everything that you do requires energy—and this is true all the way down to your cells. Your cells need excess amounts of energy because they have to keep doing their jobs 24/7. They will break down organelles and proteins that no longer help them when you deprive them of energy because they always need to find energy somewhere.

If you don't generate autophagy except when you are sleeping, a lot of negative consequences are likely—one of them being low energy. Many people who don't have much energy feel this way because their cells are not running optimally. Their cells are having to drag along all their cellular waste getting in the way. If you don't fast to force them to clean this out, they will still do it, but not nearly enough.

The mitochondria are where all of your energy starts. This is the organelle where your cell makes energy so it can perform all the jobs that it has to do. This chapter focuses on the benefits for your body, but it is useful to think about things from a microscopic point of view, too. The mitochondrion is arguably one of the most important organelle in your cells. If your mitochondrion is working well, this is a sign that your cell is working well. When scientists look at mitochondrial health in people, they find that those with well-functioning mitochondria are at low risk for neurodegenerative diseases like Huntington's, Alzheimer's, and Parkinson's.

Your mitochondria do their job best when they don't have to deal with clutter. Clutter builds up around your mitochondria in their cell from all the sources we have mentioned, and this slows it down. When you don't generate autophagy enough, this has negative consequences for mitochondria all over your body—negative consequences for the one place where all your energy ultimately comes from. It's no wonder that people who fast have more energy. Their cells' power plants are working better than they ever have before!

It is likely that you have heard of ATP before. ATP is the particle that is fundamental to your body's energy at an atomic level. ATP is where all of your cells get their energy. It doesn't matter whether your cells get energy from breaking down your food or from breaking down toxins—ATP is at the center of the process.

The details of ATP breakdown are truly fascinating, but for our purposes, we can summarize by saying that your cells use the energy that comes from converting ATP into ADP and back into ATP again (and so on). Now, this process of ATP breakdown require two things: oxygen and nourishment. All living things break down ATP, be they animals or plants. The main difference is animals use oxidation, and plants use photosynthesis.

The fascinating truth about ATP is that your system generates around 170 pounds of it each day, despite the fact that there are only around 9 ounces of ATP in your body at any given time. You only ever have half a pound of ATP in your body, yet the process of transformation of ATP gives your body energy to go through the weight of a human. The process of ATP breakdown occurs in the mitochondria of all of your cells. When you let ATP happen using toxins, dead organelles, and proteins during intermittent fasting, this makes the process much more effective.

Remember: your cells don't have brains like you do, because if they did, they would know that they should clean themselves out to make ATP breakdown happen more smoothly. But now that you know this yourself, this is no longer a problem. Make IF a regular part of your life and start seeing your energy levels spike.

Autophagy: It's What's Good for You

The fact is, not everyone thinks as much about their general health as they should. The sad thing is that once you are diagnosed with something that could have been prevented, you wish that you had thought more about taking care of your body.

If you are reading now and the good thing is that it is never too late to turn around your attitude about your health and caring for your body with the mindfulness that you should. We are primarily focused on what autophagy can do for your health through intermittent fasting, but the habits that make it more potent are the same ones that you should keep up for the betterment of your health in general.

It should be enough to tell you that intermittent fasting reduces your risk for neurodegenerative diseases. The older you get, the higher your chances of getting one of these outcomes. It is within your power to lower your risk, and these new habits don't just increase the length of your life. They make you feel better, too, and so improve the quality of your life.

We won't spend too much more time on Alzheimer's and the rest since we have already talked about them a lot, but diabetes is a disease that should not be taken lightly, either. Many people live with diabetes, but that doesn't mean it has no consequences. If you don't have it already, it is certainly worth the change in lifestyle to avoid it.

IF is a great path to staying away from diabetes. People who get this disease end up with amyloid deposits in their arteries, but if their cells had broken down the amyloid during autophagy, they likely wouldn't have gotten diabetes in the first place. Scientists are still learning more about the potential of this process to treat these diseases, but what we can already do is stop them in their tracks through intermittent fasting.

You can look at the positive effects of it on your overall health from two different angles. First and most obviously, there is the angle of stopping microbes and pathogens before they become an issue. If your body is in the mode of autophagy half the time because you are passionate about it and intermittent fasting, there is a very good chance you will rarely have to worry about infection—because your cells always deal with them very early.

Intermittent fasting spurs the biological process of autophagy that puts a stopper on many risks for age-related disease: chronic inflammation, high blood pressure, being overweight, and more. Autophagy's lowering of inflammation is often

60

underappreciated in research. Inflammation is something that can speed up the progression of disease when something else is wrong. You may have an infection, but if you have a relatively low level of inflammation, there is a good chance that your body will eventually take care of it. If you have high inflammation and you get an infection, however, the issue is compounded. Your system is sluggish and doesn't fight off the pathogen before it is too late.

The earlier you start IF, the better because your autophagy process won't be as potent at first. Even if you do everything right—paying attention to your nutrients, not consuming too many calories, exercising, drinking enough water, and following your IF regimen—your first month or so of fasting won't do nearly as much as the months after. It takes time for your body to break toxins down. If you had not ever fasted before, your autophagy is now working on a backlog of old toxins that will take time to get there. Luckily, once this is finished, it will be better than ever.

And on the subject of inflammation, once autophagy decreases your inflammation, it will be more effective as well. If you have not talked to your doctor about inflammation before, you might not be sure if yours is problematic or not. You might have high inflammation if you have bad habits like smoking, overeating, alcohol abuse, or following a sedentary lifestyle.

Some of the most recent studies about this system have shown that inadequate inflammation is a contributing factor to many neurodegenerative diseases. I have already made clear that it fights against these diseases, but now you should know precisely why. It all has to do with a special kind of it: chaperone-mediated autophagy. We will go into more detail on what this distinction means later one. This is what you need to know for now, though—biologists found that the gene instructing your cells to go through chaperone-mediated autophagy was damaged in people with neurodegenerative diseases. Since the gene was damaged, they did not go through the chaperone-mediated one when they should have. Next, proteins piled up inside the brain cells of people with these diseases. The buildup of protein gets to a point where the brain cells don't work properly anymore, and they die.

There is another theory on how it happens, but it has the same result. Other scientists think that the autophagosome (transporter essential to chaperone-mediated autophagy and macro-autophagy) binds to the lysosome (cell stomach) too strongly. As a result, there is a clogging effect, and too many proteins crowded into a cell, leading to its dysfunction and eventual death. It can be tempting to think that such things are inevitable. It can seem like you can't do anything about what happens in your brain cells. You think, just let it be. It is outside of my control. But this is not true at all. There are many people who do not ever get these diseases. Of course, we cannot deny that genes play a role, but saying that genes determine everything is just a way of not doing what we can.

Let's assume that the scientists who say neurodegeneration happens because of the "clogging effect" are right. The way you should look at it is that you can still prevent the issue from getting out of hand, just like you can with infections. When the clogging effect happens in people's brain cells, it doesn't happen in every single one.

This gives you the opportunity to generate autophagy in the cells without the clogging effect so they can clean out the protein buildups before they get out of hand. If you do this on a regular basis, you won't have to have the stress of a damaged gene.

Your cells inevitably age just like we do and get damaged genes. This doesn't mean that we should give up on them and simply allow them to not work as well as they could. Our cells without damaged DNA can pick up the slack for the ones who do. Besides, the chaperone-mediated one has another role that we have not yet gotten to. Scientists were excited to see that this special kind of process is actually responsible for repairing your cells' DNA.

If you use IF regularly—especially if you are making autophagy unleash to its fullest extent—you can even repair the genes that prevent it from working the way it should. The two methods can teach all of us to take more initiative with our health. When you learn how much control we really have, it can serve as quite a wake-up call. All you need is the knowledge of how it works and the will to live healthily for as long as possible.

Chapter 4 – The Different Types of Autophagy and they are linked to Achieving the best Intermittent Fasting Results

"The philosophy of fasting calls upon us to know ourselves, to master ourselves, and to discipline ourselves the better to free ourselves. To fast is to identify our dependencies, and free ourselves from them."
- Tariq Ramadan

At the heart of intermittent fasting's benefits is the science that makes all of it work. Autophagy is the biological process in which your cells, when unable to get energy from food, consume "junk" materials such as unused organelles, proteins, and foreign toxins.

You put your body through this biological process when you do intermittent fasting because you are depriving your cells of food to consume, so they switch to autophagy to get their energy. Because of this, you can reap all the advantages of it by simply not eating during certain windows of the day.

This will be the chapter where we dive into the biological component of intermittent fasting, one of which is the trigger of the process of autophagy. I know that science is not everyone's cup of tea, but you need to know this essential information, so you know how to best set up your IF routine.

Even if you are a fan of learning about science, it is easy to get overwhelmed with information overload, but there is a simple fact that will make things easier for you. I am not leaving out anything important in this chapter. You can rest easy knowing that you are not missing something important about autophagy in this chapter.

Part of the reason for learning the science behind intermittent fasting is so important is because you need to be certain of autophagy's significance yourself. If you can't tell your friends in a few sentences why you are doing intermittent fasting, you will lose sight of the purpose of it, and you might be in danger of stopping. You will have more than a few sentences to say to back up this science after reading this chapter. It is probable that you might annoy your friends with facts about autophagy for a week or so after reading!

They might be annoyed with you, but they won't be able to discredit the points you're making, so you will probably be doing their health a favor. Doing intermittent fasting is a lot more fun when you have friends or family doing it with you, so learning the ins and outs of the science behind it is a great opportunity to recruit others to help you live more healthily.

Now that you know the context under which it is great to know the ins and outs of the science behind intermittent fating and by extension, autophagy, we will explore the different kinds of autophagy that exist and how they apply to intermittent fasting.

Micro-autophagy

This is the form that autophagy takes in every single cell of your body. All cells have lysosomes, and those lysosomes have the chief purpose of conducting micro-autophagy. As usual, their job is to bring in damaged organelles to break them down. This is different from macro-autophagy and chaperone-mediated autophagy, where the lysosome does not pull in the cellular waste on its own. In those kinds of autophagy, a special organelle called the autophagosome has the job of finding waste inside and outside of the cell. Then, it carries them over to the lysosome and binds with it to break down its contents.

This form happens in every cell because it does some very important jobs. It helps with the homeostasis (the maintenance of the internal environment) of the membrane, and it keeps the cell's organelles at their current size.

The chemical function of the lysosome is to break down cellular waste by attacking them with enzymes. Finally, micro-autophagy is finished, and the cell uses the raw materials attained from breaking down the waste for its part of the cell cycle. The cell can use the materials for building a new cell, building a new organelle, or for building even more basic things like glucose, amino acids, fatty acids, and so forth.

Macro-autophagy

Macro-autophagy is the type of autophagy that is only seen in cells with certain jobs. This type and chaperone-mediated autophagy use the autophagosome. The autophagosome can be simply described as a vesicle. That is, it can carry things inside of it and transport them. This vesicle (the autophagosome) travels around inside the cell and goes outside the cell to find waste to break down when you are fasting, and food is scarce. When it is done wandering through the cytoplasm (the liquid environment within each cell), finding waste, it returns to the lysosome and binds with it.

When the autophagosome takes the materials into the lysosome, this is called sequestration; it has a double membrane around it that it uses to trap materials inside. When sequestration occurs, both membranes open so that the lysosome can take the toxins that the vesicle found. But in macro-autophagy, it is not the lysosome that breaks down the toxins, but the autophagosome. It can only break them down when it is bonded to the lysosome, however.

Since it only happens in specialized cells like white blood cells, there are actually a few different kinds of macro-autophagy itself, such as mitophagy and ribophagy. Most of the time, these different kinds of macro-autophagy are made for getting rid of specific organelles that have stopped working.

Chaperone-Mediated Autophagy

The direction of biology and medicine may hinge on our newest findings about this kind of autophagy: chaperone-mediated autophagy. Scientists have known about the other two types of it for much longer than chaperone-mediated autophagy. It was Yoshinori Ohsumi's research that led to the interest in it that spurred its discovery. The findings that we have so far will influence science and medicine for decades to come.

The chaperone-mediated one is the most specialized of the three types of autophagy. Essentially, this kind of autophagy differentiates itself because it uses chains of proteins to move materials into the lysosome. The proteins themselves are specialized for this one purpose in chaperone-mediated autophagy, and the materials they help move into the lysosome are specific proteins that chaperone-mediated autophagy seeks after.

In our chapter about the benefits of intermittent fasting, we went chaperone-mediated autophagy briefly because of its job of DNA repair. I am about to go into all the wonders of chaperone-mediated autophagy and what we know about it so far, but we can summarize the most important facts about chaperone-mediated autophagy briefly.

For one, it does not only break down proteins. It has a vital role in repairing DNA. As we learned earlier, the DNA repair of cells is very important because damaged DNA leads to cells not performing as they should be. When your brain cells have damaged genes, they don't perform autophagy when they should, and the result is buildups of proteins that lead to Alzheimer's, Parkinson's, and Huntington's.

Next, chaperone-mediated autophagy is important because it seeks after specific proteins to break them down. This is crucial because if chaperone-mediated autophagy did not do this, the raw materials from those proteins could be lacking in a cell, and it wouldn't be able to proceed in the cell cycle as efficiently.

Besides these two important jobs, chaperone-mediated autophagy has some others, too. Studies have concluded that chaperone-mediated autophagy plays a role in your cell metabolism and in controlling your glucose levels. Keeping your glucose relatively low is what makes autophagy possible in the first place.

Micro-autophagy and macro-autophagy might end up breaking down important proteins for the raw materials they need, but they can't use specialized protein chains to seek specific proteins out.

Cells that perform chaperone-mediated autophagy know which proteins to seek out because of the instructions from their genes. It is useful that chaperone-mediated autophagy is also needed to repair the DNA of cells because it needs that DNA to do its job.

In the last chapter, we learned that the precursor to Alzheimer's and similar diseases is damaged DNA inside cells. I told you that you shouldn't accept this as something you can't control because using autophagy; you do have the power to fight against damaged DNA and eventual neurodegeneration.

You can use this book as a life-changing resource to optimize the effects of it and repair your cell DNA as often as possible. Anything you could ever need to know about how to do this is contained in here.

While we are getting more in the weeds about the chaperone-mediated process, you should learn about the latest gene related to it: LAMP-2A. This name stands for lysosome-associated membrane protein.

We know a few things about this gene already, such as:

1. It has a strong link to chaperone-mediated autophagy
2. When scientists preserve this gene in lab mice, they had better outcomes in health and longer lifespans than mice without having this gene protected.

One scientist even noted that the mice whose LAMP-2A was protected had "healthier-looking fur" and "a glow about them."

If these symptoms sound familiar, it's because they are close to the ones that humans experience when they trigger autophagy by fasting. Your skin gets a glow, and while we don't have fur, there's a good chance the new hair you grow will be healthier, too.

When I told you that chaperone-mediated autophagy could repair DNA, regulate metabolism, and control glucose levels, all of these jobs are actually due to instructions that your cells get from their LAMP-2A gene. It's also the gene that probably gets damaged in people who develop neurodegenerative diseases.

The LAMP-2A gene is supposed to tell your specialized cells to start chaperone-mediated autophagy and seek out the specific proteins named in their DNA. When these genes are damaged, your autophagy does not function as it is supposed to, and all the biological processes that rely on it start to have problems as well.

Some of the recent findings have turned out to be incredibly relevant to matters of personal health. It has only been in the past decade that we found out that Alzheimer's and Parkinson's disease are a result of a mutation in a gene that controls autophagy.

Let's step back for a second and define what we mean by mutation. As we age, the DNA in our cells becomes damaged from wear and tear. One of the genes in our DNA is the one that controls autophagy. When that gene takes damage, our autophagy is less effective because it is not getting proper instructions from the DNA.

As a result, when your brain cells create protein chains to do certain jobs, these protein chains become clusters that are toxic to your cells, all because these cells did not have undamaged genes from which to take their instructions.

Now you might worry that this gene damage as a result of age means that there is nothing you can do about it, but this could not be further from the truth. Your takeaway from this scientific discovery should be that you need to manually turn on autophagy as you get older because your cells' genes will not be as effective at doing it automatically. You can turn on it through fasting and exercise and get the same much-needed autophagy as you would if your genes instructed your cells to do it to themselves.

Microscopic Changes Lead to Huge Consequences
Perhaps you are a reader who is skeptical about something so small having such an impact. You believe that all the science is true, but you don't think that your cells are what you should focus on when you could focus on your specific organs or certain muscles.

It might help for you to think of yourself as one big cell. As you, the cell, age, you take damage. Cells that have gone through damage do not work as well until they go through autophagy and fix their injuries.

In much the same way, you as a person can suffer injuries, and those injuries impede your ability to do what you need to do. If you got in an accident tomorrow and broke your hand, there are a lot of things you wouldn't be able to do, even if you don't have to go to work. Things that used to be simple—like getting the mail—are not simple anymore.

A cell with an injury to the mitochondria is not in the right state to cooperate with the rest of your cells. Ultimately, we are talking about just one cell here, and it doesn't do any good alone—especially if it is injured and not working properly.

It might seem like one cell does not matter much, but you have over 30 trillion cells in your whole body. That's 30,000,000,000,000 cells.

You aren't made of anything else, either. Just cells. Every one of these cells matter or they would not be in your body. Easily, an issue with one cell can spread to other cells. Health conditions arise when cells throughout your body suffer from the same issue and not getting enough of the autophagy process is one such issue.

There is even a process of programmed cell death that your cell might run if they are too damaged to help the rest of the tissue. They also might do this if they are cancerous cells; that way, they do not hurt the rest of the body.

Since autophagy disposes of cellular waste and builds new cell structures throughout all of your cells, it is your best defense against threats to your health. All of this and more happens in your microscopic cells – tiny structures that you cannot see individually. There is no real way to talk about your autophagy outside of your cells, at least when it comes to biology.

You can't do a single thing you do without your cells, so don't underestimate them. Don't underestimate the harmful effects of DNA damage in your cells and the buildup of toxins inside them, either.

As we age, our cells get less effective at their functions. They are less effective because their organelles are so. When you have a mitochondrion or another organelle that does not perform well, it is really better to break it down and make it a new mitochondrion or other organelle. Getting your cells to do this will result in better overall health for you.

However, your cells don't know this like you do. If you want them to dispose of the bad orangeades that are making them lag behind, you have to trigger autophagy by yourself. You have already learned some of the methods that people can use to do this: intermittent fasting, water fasting, a nutrient-rich diet, exercise, a hot shower, or even a sauna will do the trick.

Your cells might not take care of their poorly performing organelles if you do not use these techniques. They might continue using the same old mitochondria without even improving it. When a lot of your cells do this, you end up feeling a difference subjectively.

The health of your cells is the health of your body. You can't micromanage trillions of cells, but you can be a puppet master and manipulate them to do what you want as best as you can.

Take a broken-down vehicle as an example. You might feel emotionally attached to a car that stopped working, but that doesn't mean that you should hold onto it forever. For the first few times that it broke down, you bought the new parts and simply fixed the car. It didn't work as well as before, and it made some suspicious noises, but you like the car, so you allowed it.

But then there is the final straw. You have put thousands of dollars into the car, and at this point, even though you have an attachment to it, you can't justify spending all this money on a car that will just keep breaking down soon after you fix it.

You might say that your cells get attached to their organelles. They don't literally, of course, but they certainly won't get rid of them until they absolutely have to.

This illustrates that your cells are working in maintenance mode. When you use all of the methods to trigger advanced autophagy together, you can basically communicate with your cells, saying: "I want you to take out the trash."

Your cells need energy, and they will dig into their reserves. If you spent many years without fasting and without following a generally healthy lifestyle, there is a good chance that it will take time for your cells to break down their problematic organelles. That's because they have so many other options for energy that have stacked up over the years.

After you do intermittent fasting for enough time, though, your cells will finally run out of options and break down their mitochondria. Then, they will use the worn out parts to build new cells. You will surely feel a difference after just a week or so doing intermittent fasting, but this is why the biggest difference in energy levels will be after a longer period of time.

You have likely heard before that humans can live for three weeks or so without eating anything. Autophagy is the reason this is true. At the end of the day, it isn't "you" who has to eat, but your cells, as they keep your body alive for weeks because there is plenty already inside of you that they can consume for energy.

But it isn't only when you are starving that your cells break down this much material. Did you know that we need around 100 grams of protein each day? It sounds like a lot, but the reason the number is so high is that you actually only get about one-third of this protein from the foods that you consume.

The other two-thirds of the proteins that your body breaks down every day are protein already inside you. This is autophagy. Even before you knew what it was, it was supplying twice the volume of protein than you were consuming yourself. In other words, your cells don't just break down the protein you eat once. They break it down several times until it is eventually converted into a useful structure. When that cellular structure stops functioning in the required way, autophagy breaks it down, and it continues on and on.

Another strange thing about this microscopic phenomenon is that you don't have to do anything special to get your body to do it. It is doing it right now, and it will continue to do it for as long as you live. You didn't do anything special to harm your proteins and organelles, either—they simply accrued damage over time while you were going about your normal life.

This phenomenon is an essential biological process that will continue whether you decide to pay attention to it or not. But think about this: why would you not want to pay close attention to a process this important? A process that has been instrumental in keeping you alive to this point?

You have the option to add to the power of it by changing your way of living, such as your eating habits and your exercise habits. We all know that the older we get, the more work we have to do to make our bodies perform the way that they should. But usually, we hear this about our organs, our bones, and our muscles. For some reason, not many say this about autophagy—even though none of these systems would function without it.

The Newest Science

It can be exciting to learn about new scientific discoveries, and the newer the discoveries are, the more exciting they are. This is our final section in the chapter is about the newest findings in science underlying intermittent fasting. More accurately, it will concentrate on the newest information that there is about autophagy.

Just keep in mind that these findings are the definition of cutting-edge, meaning there is probably more information about them by the time you read this. You might want to do some research for yourself to see if anything new has been discovered. With that said, at the time of writing, these are the latest findings we have.

To begin, there is another important gene in autophagy besides the LAMP-2A gene. It is called ATG. ATG stands for autophagy-related. As the name suggests, it describes genes associated with autophagy.

The ATG gene is often discussed alongside the protein chain VPS-34. Both of them are needed to provoke autophagy and keep it regulated. While scientists protected the LAMP-2A gene from improving the overall health of mice, they found that they could get the most out of VPS-34 by altering it. The manipulation of this protein chain may be key to treating or even curing age-related diseases.

VPS-34 is an easily manipulated chain, and this makes it a great tool for biologists trying to learn more about this process. We know that the beginning of many of the diseases we are talking about is related to the deterioration of functions related to chaperone-mediated autophagy. The ability to manipulate one of the protein chains related to chaperone-mediated autophagy (VPS-34) is a phenomenal step in the right direction for everyone who wants to end diseases like cancer.

Some say that it is only a matter of time before experiments on VPS-34 lead to a new ground-breaking discovery. When that happens, medicine as we know it—especially as it relates to aging—will be totally changed.

There is one more gene you should know: the P62 gene. This gene is often attributed to the relatively long lifespan that humans have compared to other mammals.

It took time for humans to get the P62 gene in our evolution, but what does it do? Maybe you won't be surprised that it is related to chaperone-mediated autophagy. It lets our cells know when there are dangerous products that could harm them, causing them to go into a state of stress and trigger autophagy.

When scientists created genetically mutated fruit flies and gave them the P62 gene, they survived for longer than fruit flies without the P62 gene. This experiment alone should convince you of the singular potential of the scientifically well-known phenomenon.

Now that you have a strong grasp on the research for cancer and neurodegenerative diseases as it relates to autophagy, we should spend some time on another important disease: diabetes. Then, I will recommend what foods to eat when you are following a routine of intermittent fasting in the next chapter.

You might remember learning about amyloid deposits, the buildups of proteins that lead to diabetes. There is a lesson to be learned in all these cases of diseases that could be prevented with more autophagy; they are not caused by a foreign invader. They are caused by our bodies working seemingly normally—until an invisible line is crossed, and too much protein accumulates in the cells.

If there is only one takeaway you have from this science-focused chapter, it should be that increased autophagy prevents the diseases that we can't otherwise address until it's too late.

You can't tell when your proteins are crowded out your brain cells or cells anywhere else in your body. The only way you can prevent it from becoming a problem is by intermittent fasting regularly. If you do that, you will know that you are doing everything you can do to stave off diseases for which there is no other real treatment at the moment.

Chapter 5 – Diet Recommendations for Intermittent Fasting

"Fasting, or intermittent fasting, gives us an opportunity to really get all the best cells all the time and that's what we all want." - Steven Gundry

If there is one thing to remember in an intermittent fast, it's this: lower your consumption of carbohydrates. The reason for this is that carbs will be used as your body's first source of energy as long as it is present. As a result, advanced autophagy will not be triggered in its presence.

This ends up reducing the amount of time your body goes through advanced autophagy. Carbs are also the first thing your gut decides to break down—it will break down carbs before protein or fat. With that important tip in mind, let's get into the best foods to eat if you want to maximize the good your body gets from intermittent fasting.

Your general guiding principle needs to be that you have to stop eating without thinking—that is, you need to recognize the different physical and mental consequences that you will have because of the foods that you eat. Once you get really good at following this principle, all the other tips that you hear just seem like common sense.

To quickly review the food we previously told you help with autophagy, they are the reishi mushroom, turmeric, green tea, and ginger. Others are caffeine, and olive oil.

All of these foods contain chemicals that will help your body have better autophagy when you trigger it, but they will not do it alone—not without fasting or exercise. Don't get that mixed up.

There are still more foods that you might consider. Grapes have also been found to help, for example. The autophagy-trigger chemical in grapes is called Cannabidiol (CBD). CBD is the non-psychoactive brother of tetrahydrocannabinol (THC), is proved to benefit as well. CBD works particularly well for this purpose because it lessens the amount of inflammation in your body while also improving your neural connections leading the charge to autophagy.

You don't want to spend too much time thinking about what special foods to eat—at least not until you get to a point with intermittent fasting where you can trust yourself to do it without slipping. So it is best to introduce autophagy-triggering foods that you are familiar with and that are easy to access, such as those mentioned so far. After you have gained that comfort, you can introduce more exotic foods into the mix. When that happens, it can be an exciting way to mix things up.

Ultimately, eating these foods is just doing extra to make your autophagy more advanced. More important than eating these specific foods is getting a balanced diet when you are not inside your fasting window. The rest of the chapter will focus on this because it is much more important.

They say that Americans are overweight because of sugar and fats, and this is only partly true, but the true culprit is carbohydrates. Carbs are the "fluff" of nutrients—they take up a lot of space compared to others, and it is very easy to get too much of them.

Do not misinterpret this and think that you should stay away from carbs altogether. You need carbs just like you need all other nutrients. However, it is very easy to get the carbs that you need daily without even trying.

Carbs are a lot like protein this way—it isn't hard to figure out where you will get them, most of the time, because they are in a lot of the foods around us. Knowing the usual suspects that fall into the carbohydrates category gives you the advantage of knowing what to avoid to bring your carb intake down. To help you lose weight faster, burn the excess fat that you carry and to trigger autophagy most easily, you should limit your carb intake to 50g or less daily. Don't know what 50g of carbs looks like? Don't worry. Let me help you with this handy list. Food portions that contain 50g of carbs include:

- 3 slices of whole wheat bread
- 2 medium bakes sweet potatoes
- 1 ¼ medium baked potatoes
- 1 ¾ cup cooked oatmeal
- 1 cup whole grain rice
- 1 ¼ cup cooked quinoa

If you love you carbs as most people do, it is best to fill up on complex carbs rather than simple carbs. Simple carbs are food that contain a lot of sugars like raw sugar, brown sugars, fruit juice concentrate and high-fructose corn syrup. Therefore, it is best to avoid such carbohydrates. Common examples of food that contain a high amount of sugar include:

- Soda
- Packaged cookies
- Baked goods
- Breakfast cereals
- Candy
- Energy drinks

- Ice-cream

On the other hand, complex carbs pack more nutritional value and are more filling. These characteristics makes them better options for losing weight and achieving better health overall. Examples of complex carbs foods include:

- Beans
- Fiber-rich fruits
- Fiber-rich veggies
- Whole grains
- Potatoes
- Brown rice
- Quinoa

It is time for you to learn about protein cycling. Protein cycling is a diet change that many people make when they do intermittent fasting. Basically, it means alternating between days of normal protein intake and low protein intake.

It is still important that you eat a normal amount of protein on normal days because protein is an essential nutrient in your body. You need some level of normal protein every day, so your cells have it to build structures.

However, the low-protein days are important too. Having days where you consume little protein will further spur your cells to turn on the process during your fasting window.

Your cells already have plenty of protein lying around as cellular garbage, so your cells can reliably use this as their source of protein on your low-protein days. (Don't forget the fact we learned earlier—your body processes 100 grams of it each day, and only a quarter of that comes from the food you eat!)

With all that in mind, you never want to consume lots of protein, no matter how important a nutrient it is. There is a very good reason for this, as when you eat lots of protein; all you are doing is giving your cells lots of cellular garbage to clean out.

Your cells have to cycle between normal, non-stressed periods and autophagy periods, so it takes time for your cells to dispose of all of this excess.

When they take too long to do it, it eventually becomes toxic, as we have learned. Despite how essential a nutrient protein is, there is such thing as too much of a good thing.

When your diet is very high in protein, this hampers the progress of autophagy greatly. It does not hamper its progress as much as carbohydrates do, but it still slows things down. Instead of cleaning out your existing cellular garbage when you do intermittent fasting, you will simply be cleaning out the junk left behind by all the protein you just ate.

Protein cycling gives us a great chance to discuss the importance of finding a balance between IF and a healthy diet. When you do protein cycling, you still need to eat the recommended amount of protein for a reason: it is an essential nutrient.

However, you can go too far in either direction. A lot of the foods people love a diet containing a high amount of protein. So, it is common for people to eat far more protein than they should without even realizing it.

On the other hand, starving yourself of protein to the extreme is harmful, too. If you do this, you may experience loss in muscle tone that is usually associated with fasts more extreme than intermittent fasting.

To do protein cycling right, simply eat the recommended amount of protein every other day and half or less that amount on your other days.

This is not only about protein, though. Even though intermittent is a fast meant for everyone, there are still ways we can take it too far. Take someone who makes their fasting window too long: let's say, 14 hours. That would mean they eat for an hour in the morning and then eat again for an hour before bed. This is absolutely unhealthy, and I strongly recommend avoiding it.

I especially advise against it because the intermittent fasting is meant to be done every day. If you are fasting for 14 hours every day, that could have serious consequences on your body. With water fast, you may fast for as much as 24 or 48 hours, but the difference is the frequency. Someone can do a water fast all day on Sunday and then go back to their normal eating patterns on Monday.

But if they do intermittent for 14 hours a day, there is never a time they return to their regular eating pattern. Their regular eating pattern involves consuming far too infrequently.

Maybe you are familiar with the concept of yin and yang from Taoism. The yang gives, and the yin takes. To find a balance between a healthy diet and intermittent fasting, keep thinking of eating as yang and IF as yin. You need yang to fill yourself up with fresh nutrients. When you are following it, you do this outside of your fasting window. You need yin to cleanse your cells of the toxins produced from yang.

Too much of yang (eating) and too much of yin (fasting) both have negative consequences. The key is to find a balance between the two; this will allow you to get the benefits of both.

Put another way; don't let yourself believe that "extra" fasting will lead to better health outcomes. It won't. If you truly want to be healthy, you need to find the right about eating for your yang and the right amount of fasting for your yin.

Even a cup of coffee at the beginning of your fast period can mess things up. Don't take the risk when you are already looking to get as much as possible out of autophagy.

Another common mistake is consuming flavored water during the fast period. Do not do this—again, the flavoring has something that your body has to break down. When your body breaks down chemicals, autophagy stops. You should even stay away from smells of flavor. It sounds bizarre, but even the smell of real or artificial food causes a parasympathetic reaction from your vagus nerve.

This reaction will actually keep autophagy from happening to a significant degree because it stimulates mTOR, a gene that will stop it when activated. It may feel like there is such a delicate balance, but if you are intermittent fasting to maximize the potential of it, these are the things you have to consider.

Don't even take vitamins or supplements that purport to boost autophagy during your period of fast. Not to beat a dead horse, but: your body has to process that, and then it won't start until it's done.

People who advocate for these supplements say that supplements don't have enough digestible chemicals to stop this method from happening, but they don't really know this is the case. They are just selling a supplement. (On a side note, there is no official supplement that is known to turn on or even aid the method at this moment, so you shouldn't bother shopping around for them.)

The list of what to avoid goes on. If it doesn't occur naturally and it comes in colorful packaging, stay away from it. Don't drink soda, eat candy, or buy any of the meat from your grocery store that comes from factory farms. All the nutrients you should be indirectly getting from the grass that animal ate is not there, because these animals are stuffed with chemicals instead of fed grass.

It should probably go without saying, but you need to stay away from sugar even when it is not the sweet stuff on your kitchen counter. Ideally, most of the sugars in your diet come from fruits, and you don't even want to eat too many of those. Even eating more than a little bit of fruit can put too much sugar into your system, so that should tell you how bad sugar is for you.

Artificial sugars are especially dangerous and you simply don't need them. When you consume artificial sugar, you are adding a lot of waste that your cells will have to clean out later.

In fact, this is the image that you should conjure with all of the foods you put into your system. Imagine your broken-down, microscopic foods inside your cells. What will be the most useful to your cells (again, your cells make up all of you): sugary foods or foods with tons of vitamins?

We all know the answer, but the harder part is following through. Actually, doing it may not be as hard as you think. Once you have made the decision to start intermittent fasting day, you should go grocery shopping. This is what makes it easy: all you have to do is refrain from buying the foods that we are talking about.

Don't buy bagels. Don't buy packaged snacks. Don't buy the cake mix.

Instead, put dairy products in your cart, those have healthy protein. Put in some natural fruit juice and cucumbers. Pick up healthy nuts like cashews. Find a recipe that you think looks tasty and uses the foods that you want to take part of your normal diet.

Recipes are the key to changing your diet. This is for many reasons. You will also feel good about making food at home, and saving money by not going out to eat.

Going out to eat is a big risk, particularly in the early stages of intermittent fasting. I advise you not to go out to eat until you can at least keep yourself from eating during your fast for two weeks.

Now, let's get right to it. What should you be eating when you do the intermittent?

First and foremost: water. Every system that keeps you alive needs water to keep going, and that doesn't stop being true when you are fasting. The color of your urine will tell you if you are drinking enough water. The clearer it is, the better— although if it is totally clear, that means you are drinking too much water. There is a limit to the amount of water you should drink every day. It depends on your weight and height and exceeding that amount can lead to you essentially drowning your cells.

Another boon of drinking a lot of water during intermittent fasting is that it keeps your cravings away. A lot of times, we think that we want food, but what we really feel is thirst.

Next, you need to make fish a weekly dish. They are your best source of Omega-3 fats, an important nutrient for autophagy to occur. Fish also have vitamins and protein. The American Heart Association tells us we should be eating at least one serving of fish every week. Are you?

Potatoes are a good food option, too. They are especially filling, while actually giving us real nutrients. Getting full on potatoes will keep you from eating when you are supposed to be fasting. There is even research showing that people with potatoes in their diets have more success in losing weight.

We will put legumes and beans in the same category, as most people think of them as the same thing, anyway. Beans are a notably good source of energy while somewhat paradoxically being low in calories. Much like potatoes, beans have been shown to be part of diets where people succeeded in losing weight.

You might already know this, but you still have to be somewhat careful with beans and legumes because they are high in carbs. But I still say they are good for intermittent fasting for all the reasons listed.

Now we are on to the nuts. What makes this a great option is that they have unsaturated fats: the kind that you want. Specifically, nuts have polyunsaturated fats, just like olive oil. Walnut is one example of a food with this healthy fat. You don't have to worry about the calories for nuts either, because, for the healthy ones like walnuts, they usually end up being insignificant.

I don't want to spend too much time on vegetables because everyone knows that we are supposed to eat vegetables, but I will give you one more reason to eat them: they are packed with fiber. Of course, fiber aids in digestion. When you combine your fiber from your vegetable-rich diet with intermittent fasting, your digestive system will be as healthy as it can be. Fiber is also great for intermittent fasting because it keeps you from feeling hungry during your fasting periods.

Avocados seem to be quite popular these days, but they really should be with intermittent fasting practitioners. They are considered a "superfood" because they have a lot of the vitamins and nutrients that you need every day. Best of all, they have unsaturated fats. You can start eating a lot of avocados and get a lot of what you need from them so you can lower your caloric consumption.

While green tea may have chemicals that directly influence the power of autophagy, other teas could help with aspects of intermittent fasting from a more pragmatic standpoint. For instance, while caffeine has been shown to help increase autophagy when it is generated, if you get that caffeine from coffee, it will also help you feel fuller. Coffee or any kind of tea may have this effect on you.

Eat eggs, too. They have the protein that you need without a lot of the unhealthy stuff that tends to come with protein. And while we are talking about studies, there is research showing that people who replace a bagel with an egg feel fewer feelings of hunger during the day—so you might want to get into the habit of eating an egg every morning so you can have the best chances of succeeding with IF.

There you have it—the foods to eat and to leave out when you do intermittent fasting. You can always check this chapter again if you're unsure what to do.

Beware the tricks your mind will play on you to make you think that you are hungry for foods that do not even have essential nutrients. You can be sure this is just your brain trying to get the food you crave into your mouth.

Many people start the very first few hours into an intermittent fast and are convinced that they are already low on energy. True fatigue is one thing, but feeling a little tired after not eating for a couple of hours doesn't mean you need to eat a meal right away. You have to let feelings like this pass, or else they will seriously hinder your fast.

You are bound to feel like you are "slightly hungry" during your time doing the intermittent fasting, especially when you first begin this journey. This is something that you should expect with any fast after you spend your whole life, never even contemplating it. Be prepared for the initial feelings and through the strength of your determination, you will defeat these feelings.

Chapter 6 – Intermittent Fasting and Women

"The reason for fasting is to understand the relationship between what's you and what's the accumulative body." - Jaggi Vasudev

There is good reason to learn about intermittent fasting specifically as it applies to women because research has demonstrated that it has different effects on men and women. Some women experienced less-than-desirable outcomes as a result of intermittent fasting. I tell you this to caution you about doing intermittent fasting in a healthy way, not to scare you from doing something that would be good for your body. Intermittent fasting needs to be practiced the right way for it to be effective and not have dire health consequences.

Some women said their menstrual cycle altered because of it, and some said their blood sugar went too low. Both of these outcomes can be avoided by consuming adequate nutrients when you are not in the fasting period of intermittent fasting and by limiting your fasting times to reasonable windows.

All the success that women have been having with intermittent fasting is the reason that it has gotten so popular suddenly. It's a pattern of eating that speaks to the health concerns that women are worried about: weight loss, risk of heart disease, risk of diabetes, and even risk of cancer.

While any person can do it, you know that women have their own specific issues that make their experience with intermittent fasting different. But how exactly do their experiences differ?

It is just one study on laboratory mice, but there is one that showed that female mice who did concurrent day fasting for 3-6 had ovaries that were shrunk and irregular cycles, too.

There is a link between the menstrual cycle and how it can interact with changes in diet in all mammalian species. There has not been any scientific backing yet on if intermittent fasting can really affect your period, but there has definitely been a limited number of cases where women say their cycles were different, and they thought that intermittent fasting was the cause.

It is hard to say if we can blame this entirely on the intermittent fasting routine itself, though. Some have suggested that since women who do it often want to lose weight, they are more likely to be overweight or obese. Being overweight or obese is a risk factor for having irregular periods, so perhaps this is the cause of the irregular cycle. However, we can't jump to conclusions.

But the menstrual cycle is not the only thing that women have to consider when doing intermittent fasting that men don't. Their hormones are also different and affect their eating habits differently.

These hormone differences give some credence to the idea that this diet can have negative consequences for women if they are not careful. The main hormone in the spotlight is GnRH, which is affected when women consume fewer calories.

If women consume too few calories, their GnRH production might be altered, which could put them at risk for irregular periods.

We do have to keep in mind that this is a side effect of low caloric intake, not intermittent fasting. Women who want to lose weight, to some extent, do have to consume fewer calories. These women may accept the temporary changes to their period, knowing that their weight loss will have many positive, long-lasting benefits.

There may still be something to the idea that women should think about their specific issues when choosing to do this diet. They might choose to intermittent fast for a shorter period of time and for fewer days.

If we are being honest, while anyone can do an intermittent fast to get the health benefits of autophagy, most of the people who are doing it are women. The science showing women some of the woman-specific problems that come with it shouldn't scare them from doing it. They should keep doing it anyway because the initial discomfort is worth the payoff they will get when they lose weight, have better skin, and have a detoxified system.

Doctors know that women have reproductive systems that are closely related to their metabolisms. This makes sense because when women are carrying children, they have to be able to feed them from the inside.

Even if you aren't pregnant, however, the deep entanglement between the female reproductive system and the female metabolism affects your body. When you have not had a period for a while during the same time that you changed your pattern of eating, there is a greater-than-luck chance that your missing period is because of your changed pattern of eating.

You don't want to give up on fasting just because it can be a little harder as a woman. Women are pros at handling adversity and coming out the winner. You need to take the challenge and do the thing that is good for your body, even when it puts you through some periods of discomfort.

Remember that hormone changes are fleeting, so if you experience a change in hormones during the time that you fast, it doesn't mean that the fast is bad for you. Over time, these hormone level will adjust until it is just another part of your day.

Getting used to it will be heightened by managing your stress and sleep. Mostly, you want to pay attention to your stress, but your stress is connected to a whole list of things. They include not eating enough calories, not getting enough nutrients, not being active enough, chronic inflammation, and finally, sleep deprivation.

If you can manage all of these things, your hormones should not give you too much of a trouble as you transition into intermittent fasting.

Nonetheless, going for an extended period of time without a period could be a sign of something serious. If this happens, you should stop your fast and schedule a doctor's visit.

Are Intermittent Fasting and Women Made for Each Other?

Don't let the anecdotal stories about irregular cycles make you afraid of doing what will ultimately be good for you. In all truth, autophagy is a wonderful way that women can take control of their bodies. Every woman on Earth wants a sustainable way to lose weight, increase muscle mass, and rev up their energy. Women that generate autophagy with intermittent fasting come with all of these rewards, so it's no wonder so many women are talking about it.

As you know well, autophagy also confers long-term health benefits, but some of them are particularly important to women: a more acute stress response from their cells so that it is easier to trigger in the future, improved sensitivity to insulin, and an increase in the growth hormone, which is vital to many processes that your body goes through.

With all of these positives from IF, it wouldn't be wise to completely ignore them due to low chances of some of the indications that it can interfere with the female reproductive system. But that only means we need to be measured in the way we generate autophagy. It doesn't mean we abandon intermittent fasting altogether.

If you ever experience any signs that this eating pattern has influenced your cycle, then it might be a good idea to avoid that longer periods of a fast. It might be better for you to fast for around 8 hours instead.

Since you don't yet know how your body will react to intermittent fasting as a woman until you have done it, I also advise you to start with a smaller fasting window with your first fast. You probably should not even fast for two days in a row during your first week, if you really want to be careful.

There are some groups of women that should not do intermittent fasting altogether. If you have had a history of problems with any major organs, such as your lungs, heart, or liver, you should not do it. It could put too much stress on these organs, and the potential benefit you would get from it would not be enough to justify you harming them.

It should be obvious that pregnant women should not fast. As I have said, the female reproductive system is closely tied to the woman's metabolism. When that woman is with child, she doesn't have the luxury of purposefully depriving herself of nutrients to generate autophagy anymore, because now the health of her body and of her child is what determines her health the most.

Sadly, there are many women with eating disorders compared to men. Women who have or who have had eating disorders should not attempt to do intermittent fasting. They are at too high a risk of losing any progress they might have made in establishing normal eating patterns.

My final two tips for women who do it are the same ones I have said throughout our book: drink a lot of water and exercise. Both of these activities will keep your body in shape so it can handle the stress of autophagy and intermittent fasting better.

Chapter 7 – Intermittent Fasting for Women over 50

"Most cultures traditionally link food and spirituality directly with periodic restrictions and celebrations punctuating the year. Abstinence from particular foods or full-on fasting is part of many religious traditions and holidays." - Marcus Samuelsson

Overweight women over 50 have a higher risk of developing diabetes and heart problems than they did when they were younger. Intermittent fasting is one option they have to manage their weight and control these increased health risks.

The metabolism of a woman over 50 has become slower, so you can't expect as quick results if you are a member of this group, but you will probably get the most out of it compared to any other group of women because of all the anti-aging effects of intermittent fasting and autophagy.

Overweight and obese people have higher risks of heart disease, stroke, and more as they age. On the other hand, people with lower BMIs are not looking at these same risks.

Losing weight can only be good for your body, and autophagy is the healthiest and most effective way to do it, as it will help you manage your weight effectively, feel good, and be healthy for years and years.

But, so far, we have only talked about the health benefits that are immediately obvious. There is a reduction of health risks that are not cosmetic, like youthful skin and weight loss but it has also been proven that an increase in the aforementioned phenomenon reduces your risk of developing Alzheimer's and Parkinson's disease. Furthermore, it also reduces inflammation, which will increase your overall health.

The chances of developing cancer increasing with age. There has even been researches about the benefits for cancer patients undergoing chemotherapy. Studies have shown that cancer patients going through chemotherapy saw a reduction in the clumps of dead white blood cells that accumulate because of it. Dead cells can be hazardous to your body if they are not cleaned out during autophagy.

Since these patients fasted in order to turn on autophagy, their bodies were able to clean out the white blood cells and recover from chemotherapy sooner.

You can only imagine the kind of advantage you get if you are turning it on as much as possible, and you aren't even looking at a major health risk yet. You may not have as big an accumulation of dead cells as someone going through chemotherapy, but if you have not fasted before and you don't exercise regularly, it is very likely that you have a lot of toxins in your body.

There are many misconceptions about how the process does its anti-aging work. Perhaps the most common is that its only health benefits come from taking care of toxins. Clearing toxins from your system is certainly a good thing, but it goes far beyond ridding your body of harmful chemicals.

Most of these toxins are not from outside your body, but they are materials like proteins and organelles that your cells used once and then no longer had a use for. These discarded materials start to take up space over time, creating clutter that slows down your cells. This is when they become toxins.

Some of these toxins cause even worse problems than congestion. The worst case is protein clusters that form in the brain. Neurodegenerative diseases like Alzheimer's become more of a concern as we age, and autophagy might be your best ally in fighting against your risk of these diseases.

From a broader perspective, Alzheimer's manifests as "knots" and "tangles" in the brain that impair memory.

When doctors look at the knots and tangles with a microscope, they see that these irregularities are actually clusters of proteins that have built up over time. They are proteins that brain cells used at one point but later had no purpose. The protein clusters were not managed with autophagy, so they simply accumulated and started leading to serious memory problems.

Alzheimer's disease is one of the most extreme consequence that you can have from not going through enough autophagy. It is not the only consequence, however. Discarded materials like protein clusters start to build up throughout your body, not just your brain, if you rarely go through this process.

In this regard, low autophagy leads to a low count of collagen, the protein that makes your skin youthful. Your skin cells can't produce collagen when they are crowded by cellular garbage. This is why loose skin is commonly associated with aging.

Similarly, you lose more muscle mass if you rarely go through it because you are not turning on it to repair the muscle tissue damage that results from physical activity.

From these examples alone, you can see that this phenomenon is more than a toxin-cleaning agent for women over 50, as it doesn't only destroy the bad (toxins); it builds the good (new organelles, proteins, and cells). Both sides of it make it such a powerful anti-aging tool, one that was surprisingly given to us by nature.

So far, we have established that it isn't just good for destroying pathogen invaders—it also destroys materials that become toxic when they linger in the cells for too long. In short, this biological process cleans out toxins from the outside and inside.

In the third stage, your cells use these broken-down parts as ingredients to build new cells and cell structures. What's more: your cells have more room to build new cells and new cell parts because they freed up so much space during autophagy.

All these things come together when you find a way to turn on it on a regular basis. Equipped with all this information, you know much more about this than even your average fasting practitioner.

Women over 50 certainly still want to manage their weight and have good skin, but it is around this age that we start to get a more mature perspective on life, and we care more about the health consequences of our daily life choices than before. They have many options for unlocking autophagy even further than they would with intermittent fasting alone.

Back in the 90s, the idea of caloric restriction became very popular, and people saw improvements in their health from doing nothing more than eating less. There is even a great deal of evidence that mammals who restrict their calories live longer than mammals who do not.

We have heard a lot of ideas about losing weight from nutritionists in the last few decades, but let's not kid ourselves: the main reason for weight gain across the planet comes down to people consuming a lot of calories without physically exerting themselves to burn them off. Fasting for any length of time will lead to consuming fewer calories, so you are on the right track for losing weight when you fast.

If you do not recycle your body's toxins by turning on autophagy regularly, your body will be over-encumbered with cellular garbage, and you will be less healthy as a result. If this analogy were expanded, you might even live a shorter life if you do not regularly clean out your cellular garbage.

Your cells try to live longer by using this method to combat their cellular aging—you should try to use autophagy to work against aging too.

Chapter 8 – Intermittent Fasting Techniques: 16/8, Keto Diet, and More

"Periodic fasting can help clear up the mind and strengthen the body and the spirit." - Ezra Taft Benson

16/8 Fasting

After talking a little bit about the different ways that women of all ages can do intermittent fasting, now it's time to go into them in more detail. The first one, and maybe the most well-known, is the 16/8 one.

The fundamental aspect of intermittent fasting—not eating for some period of the day—is easily observed in 16/8. You only eat for 8 hours of the day, and you fast for the other 16 hours. It is also typical for practitioners to follow the keto diet, the low-carb diet designed to induce ketosis in your body to help in burning body fat.

Many women get confused about what intermittent fasting requires of them because they are used to following diets, not fasts. It is a new pattern of eating, not a diet. There are foods that you should eat in an intermittent fasting since they help with the goal of autophagy, as we learned in Chapter 5. But is not a diet itself.

The other side of that is a woman thinking they can eat anything since it is not a diet. This is obviously not true either.

In one sense, intermittent fasting is simpler than dieting. You could say it's simpler because you are not basing all of your health and body goals on eating certain foods and restricting others. On a fundamental level, the most important thing to do is to commit to not eating for a number of hours at the same time every day.

But you could also say that it is more complicated because intermittent fasting alone will do everything. It needs the backing of a commitment to practicing healthy habits that will aid the overall sustenance and maintenance of good health of mind and body. The truth is, intermittent fasting does much of the work, but you will only see the results if you adopt habits that are good for your health, too.

That said, I hope this book has given you a good sense of how autophagy ties into all aspects of health, because it really does tie into intermittent fasting, working out, and eating healthy.

The point we are trying to come to is that you could work out every day and eat all of the foods you are supposed to eat, but not fast; you would be healthy, without a doubt. But on balance, you probably wouldn't be as healthy as someone who worked out a little less, ate a little less healthy, but did intermittent fasting every day.

That's because autophagy is the vital cellular process your whole body relies upon, but that people do not pay nearly enough attention to.

You are nearing the end of the book, and that means it's time to put together your plan of attack for this fast. What method of intermittent fasting are you going to do? Whichever one you choose, you should write down your exact goal for the number of hours you want to fast and the date you will start.

When the day comes, mark the actual time you start fasting and the actual time you stop. Write down whether you "cheat" during your fasting window or not. Keeping a log like this will make it a lot more likely for you to do it successfully. You can include a number of other items in this log, such as how you feel mentally, emotionally and physically, how hunger (if your experience the feeling) affected you and how you managed the different things that you felt. This journal not only give you a count of how you are doing but also allows you a means of reflection to see how far you have come.

The 12-Hour Fast

This intermittent fast is a good one to start with, although if the idea of fasting is completely new to you and makes you nervous, you are totally free to reduce it to 10 hours or less.

The trick for a simple intermittent fast like this is to ensure you are still getting a healthy number of calories every day but to simply get them outside of the 12-hour-long window that you have decided to fast for.

The 12-hour fast is also a good place to start for someone who wants to end up doing a more ambitious fast. You don't start so low that going as high as 16 hours seems infeasible.

The times during which you use the indicated approach are entirely up to you. Any approach is best done by waking up relatively early, eating breakfast, fasting, and then eating dinner. You don't want to eat too close to your bedtime because then you will be spending a lot of your precious autophagy time during sleep by breaking down your food.

It is surprising that we have not even had the opportunity to talk about the importance of sleep with autophagy. There are some facts about sleep, and you need to seriously consider it.

You do the most autophagy that you do throughout your day when you are sleeping. Even in people who do not think about fasting or autophagy whatsoever, their highest level of it is when they are sleeping, and so is yours.

That means when you eat really close to the time you go to bed—let's say you eat at 7 pm and then sleep at 9 pm—you aren't giving your body enough time to break down your food. You don't have any significant incentive to trigger autophagy when you are digesting, so digesting in your sleep is a big wasted opportunity.

Even though the 12-hour fast can prove challenging, because you don't want to wake up too unreasonably early, but you don't want to digest food during the time that you should be going through advanced autophagy while you are asleep, either.

You may choose to wake up and eat your first meal at 7 am. 12 hours later, your fast is over, and you eat dinner at 7 pm. You can probably already see how this can be problematic; if you get enough sleep to wake up at 7 am, you will want to be in bed by 10 pm. However, this does leave 3 hours between your dinner and your bedtime, so while it is a tight squeeze, this system does work out for the 12-hour fast.

The 8-Hour Fast
You could call this a beginner fast. That doesn't mean that it's a small feat, though. Don't forget that intermittent fasting is every day. 8 hours may not seem like a long time to go without food, but if you haven't done it before, doing it every day might end up being a lot harder than you expected.

Some call the 16-hour fast the "16:8 diet," so you can call this one the "8:16 diet," if you like. As you can see, leaving plenty of time between dinner and sleep is a lot easier with this eating pattern. You can eat dinner at 6 pm, go to bed at 10 pm, wake up at 7 am and get your nutrients between then and 10 am. But between 10 am and 6 pm, you are doing your intermittent fast.

104

The 5:2 Fast

Not every kind of intermittent fasting is based around the number of hours you fast every day. In earnest, I recommend doing the traditional 8-hour fast to start out and simply make it longer as you become more comfortable. However, I have said throughout the book that you have the freedom to do whatever works for you and your body—so it would be a disservice to you if I didn't let you know what other options are out there for intermittent fasting.

In 5:2, you eat the way you would normally for five days of the week (still eating healthy, though). During the other two days, women only consume 500 calories.

The usual guidance applies—you don't get to glut out on your non-fasting days just because you aren't in a fast. You will want to make sure you get all the nutrients you need on the non-fasting days, though, because you won't be able to cram many important ones into 500 calories on those days.

There are some people who think 5:2 would work better for them because they can't imagine committing to fasting every single day of the week. With 5:2, you do an extreme fast for two days of the week so that you don't have to fast at all on most days of the week.

Concurrent Day Fasting

This kind of fast itself has different versions to it, but they all follow the basic idea of fasting every other day instead of every single day. It is similar to the 5:2 fast, except you don't have to go as extreme on your fasting days.

Concurrent-day fasting, sometimes called "alternate-day fasting," has been tested in some studies, and people did have luck in losing weight when following it. The main drawback of it is that people say they never feel entirely full when following it.

If you want to follow concurrent day fasting yourself, you don't have to do much to plan it out. Of course, you eat on whatever schedule you normally would on your non-fasting days, and then every other day you fast.

Since you aren't fasting every day, you need to consider that when deciding how long you will go. You don't want to do an 8-hour fast, because that is too short, considering that you will go back to not fasting the next day. A 12 or 16-hour fast might work, depending on your experience with it so far.

You have no shortage of options for intermittent fasting. I hope you feel that thanks to this book, you are at no shortage of information, either.

You may feel somewhat overwhelmed after reading guide to intermittent fasting that is so chockfull of information. The Table of Contents may be helpful to you in case you think you should revisit a topic again.

Conclusion

Thank you for making it through to the end of *Intermittent Fasting for Women 101*, let's hope it was informative and able to provide you with all of the tools you need to achieve your goals whatever they may be.

After being exposed to so much knowledge about intermittent fasting, you aren't likely to be surprised by the fact that the American Heart Association recommends it for losing weight. Its effectiveness in helping women lose weight is backed by science as well as by the personal experiences of thousands of women.

Fasting has existed in religious traditions for millennia, and now anyone can harness its health benefits with intermittent fasting. You don't have to undergo nearly the level of physical and mental fatigue of traditional water fasts, but you still see the difference in your waistline and in how you feel.

The scientific credibility that intermittent fasting has is all thanks to the biological process of autophagy. Autophagy is your body's natural means of getting rid of toxins that pollute your system. Intermittent fasting is your means of triggering this vital process.

Biologists have been studying autophagy and its revelatory implications for health heavily in the last ten years—and some of the most important findings have been in just the last few years! Be sure to check out the appendix at the end of the book so you can learn more about what scientists are finding out.

The more and more mainstream attention that autophagy has been receiving can be attributed to the research of Nobel Prize-winning Yoshinori Ohsumi. He is the scientist who studied it in yeast cells for decades and was finally recognized for his important work.

His research led to more scientists studying the role of this process in fighting cancer and age-related disease. What has been found is that triggering it on purpose can help us live healthier lives, longer lives, and more youthful lives.

Intermittent fasting is your ticket into triggering autophagy because it is easy to sustain once you understand the science. Unlike other means of achieving autophagy, intermittent fasting doesn't ask that you go to the gym or change what you eat (although you should know still these things to get the most out of the biological process). Start your intermittent fast today, and you will see all the health benefits uncovered in this book for yourself.

If you're still skeptical, make sure to peruse the appendix, which is filled with scientific studies on intermittent fasting done by experts.

Finally, if you found this book useful in any way, a review on Amazon is always appreciated!

Lara Moore

Appendix
Studies on Intermittent Fasting and Autophagy

Anton, Moehl, Donahoo, Marosi, Lee, et al. *Flipping the Metabolic Switch: Understanding and Applying Health Benefits of Fasting.* 2017 Oct 31. ncbi.nlm.nih.gov/pmc/articles/PMC5783752/

This study focuses on the physical effects of intermittent fasting on the most important organs of the body. The authors conclude that lowering the level of glucose in your body can actually aid in keeping your muscle mass. They say this can be a boon for people who are struggling with their weight. They even conclude that fasting results in the activation of neural pathways with a lot of great effects, including fighting aging and slow the progression of the disease.

Bartosz, Zalewska, Wesierska, Sokolowska, et al. *Intermittent Fasting in Cardiovascular Disorders—An Overview.* Published 2019 Mar 20. ncbi.nlm.nih.gov/pmc/articles/PMC6471315/

The authors conclude that doing intermittent fasting greatly reduces the risk of getting a cardiovascular disease. Participants in this eating pattern are able to maintain a source of energy through fatty acids and ketones while the body goes through metabolic switching between glucose and ketones. These scientists even conclude that intermittent fasting helps people lose body mass by changing the transformations of your lipids. They also say that it reduces cholesterol in its practitioners.

Antunes, Erustes, Costa, Nascimento, et al. *Autophagy and intermittent fasting: the connection for cancer therapy?* Published 2018 Nov 27. ncbi.nlm.nih.gov/pmc/articles/PMC6257056/

These authors examine the role that autophagy can play in fighting against cancer. They write that this phenomenon can either help cancer cells grow or help non-cancerous cells grow to fight against them, depending on the situation. They consider the possible use of autophagy for fighting tumors. Fasting in particular, is outlined as the chief strategy in using autophagy to fight cancer. The main conclusion is the use of it for protecting non-cancerous cells from toxic cancer cells as well as for reducing the side effects from chemotherapy.

Ganesan, Habboush, Sultan. *Intermittent Fasting: The Choice for a Healthier Lifestyle.* Published online 2018 Jul 9. ncbi.nlm.nih.gov/pmc/articles/PMC6128599/

A meta-analysis of studies done in the past 20 years on the subject of intermittent fasting. Not only did these studies show that people who did intermittent fasting lost weight, but they also improved on important biological measures like reduced low-density lipoprotein and triglyceride. No matter the body type of the studies' participants, they succeeded in losing weight on average.

Harvie, Howell. *Potential Benefits and Harms of Intermittent Energy Restriction and Intermittent Fasting Amongst Obese, Overweight and Normal Weight Subjects—A Narrative Review of Human and Animal Evidence.* Published 2017 Jan 19. ncbi.nlm.nih.gov/pmc/articles/PMC5371748/

These authors go over and compare experiments on intermittent fasting and intermittent energy restriction (referred to in this book as a caloric restriction). Their findings are that there is no real evidence of either method being harmful, and while both methods show promise for helping people lose weight, fasting is more consistently effective. They note that there is a lack of research on the effective of intermittent fasting and caloric restriction on people who are not overweight or obese.

Jacomin, Gul, Sudhakar, Korcsmaros, Nezis. *What We Learned from Big Data for Autophagy Research*. Published 2018 Aug 17. ncbi.nlm.nih.gov/pmc/articles/PMC6107789/

The scientists went into this study wanting to investigate the relation between autophagy and other integral cellular processes. They use big data to do an overview of what biologists have learned about this relation. The authors find that autophagy plays an important part in many different pathologies, including in infections and in cancer. Its role in neurodegenerative diseases is also well-known.

Yoshii, Mizushima. *Monitoring and Measuring Autophagy*. 2017 Sep 18. ncbi.nlm.nih.gov/pmc/articles/PMC5618514/

Yoshii and Mizushima examine a number of Meta-issues in studying autophagy, including the use of mice and their anatomical closeness to humans and the accuracy of the results in studies that use samples to make conclusions about autophagy in human beings.